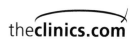

NURSING CLINICS
OF NORTH AMERICA

Holistic Nursing

GUEST EDITOR
Noreen Frisch, PhD, RN, FAAN, APHN

CONSULTING EDITOR
Suzanne S. Prevost, PhD, RN

June 2007 • Volume 42 • Number 2

SAUNDERS

An Imprint of Elsevier, Inc.
PHILADELPHIA   LONDON   TORONTO   MONTREAL   SYDNEY   TOKYO

W.B. SAUNDERS COMPANY
A Division of Elsevier Inc.

1600 John F. Kennedy Blvd., Suite 1800, Philadelphia, PA 19103-2899

http://www.theclinics.com

NURSING CLINICS OF NORTH AMERICA
June 2007
Editor: Ali Gavenda

Volume 42, Number
ISSN 0029-64•
ISBN-13: 978-1-4160-4342
ISBN-10: 1-4160-4342•

The ideas and opinions expressed in *Nursing Clinics of North America* do not necessarily reflect those of t• Publisher. The Publisher does not assume any responsibility for any injury and/or damage to persons property arising out of or related to any use of the material contained in this periodical. The reader is a vised to check the appropriate medical literature and the product information currently provided by t manufacturer of each drug to be administered to verify the dosage, the method and duration of admin tration, or contraindications. It is the responsibility of the treating physician or other health care profsional, relying on independent experience and knowledge of the patient, to determine drug dosages a the best treatment for the patient. Mention of any product in this issue should not be construed as endor ment by the contributors, editors, or the Publisher of the product or manufacturers' claims.

Nursing Clinics of North America (ISSN 0029-6465) is published quarterly by Elsevier Inc., 360 Park Aven• South, New York, NY 10010-1710. Months of issue are March, June, September, and December. Busin• and Editorial Offices: 1600 John F. Kennedy Blvd., Suite 1800, Philadelphia, PA 19103-2899. Customer S vice Office: 6277 Sea Harbor Drive, Orlando, FL 32887-4800. Periodicals postage paid at New York, N and additional mailing offices. Subscription price per year is, $116.00 (US individuals), $216.00 (US ins tutions), $187.00 (international individuals), $259.00 (international institutions), $160.00 (Canadian indi duals), $259.00 (Canadian institutions), $61.00 (US students), and $94.00 (international students). To rece• student/resident rate, orders must be accompanied by name of affiliated institution, date of term, and t signature of program/residency coordinator on institution letterhead. Orders will be billed at individ• rate until proof of status is received. Foreign air speed delivery is included in all *Clinics* subscription pric All prices are subject to change without notice. **POSTMASTER:** Send address changes to *Nursing Clin* Elsevier Periodicals Customer Service, 6277 Sea Harbor Drive, Orlando, FL 32887-4800. **Customer Servi** **1-800-654-2452 (US). From outside of the US, call 1-407-345-4000.**

Nursing Clinics of North America is covered in *EMBASE/Excerpta Medica, Index Medicus, Social Sciences C• tion Index, Current Contents, ASCA, Cumulative Index to Nursing, RNdex Top 100,* and *Allied Health Literat• and International Nursing Index (INI).*

Printed in the United States of America.

CONSULTING EDITOR

SUZANNE S. PREVOST, PhD, RN, Nursing Professor and National HealthCare Chair of Excellence, Middle Tennessee State University, School of Nursing, Murfreesboro, Tennessee

GUEST EDITOR

NOREEN FRISCH, PhD, RN, FAAN, APHN, Professor and Director, School of Nursing, Cleveland State University, Cleveland, Ohio

CONTRIBUTORS

CHERYL DELGADO, PhD, RN, ANP-BC, Assistant Professor, School of Nursing, Cleveland State University, Cleveland, Ohio

JOAN ENGEBRETSON, DrPH, AHN-BC, RN, Professor, Department of Target Populations, School of Nursing, University of Texas Health Science Center–Houston, Houston, Texas

HELEN L. ERICKSON, PhD, RN, AHN-BC, FAAN, Professor Emeritus, Holistic Adult Nursing, The University of Texas at Austin; and Board of Directors and Chair, American Holistic Nurses Certification Corporation, Cedar Park, Texas

NOREEN FRISCH, PhD, RN, FAAN, APHN, Professor and Director, School of Nursing, Cleveland State University, Cleveland, Ohio

MARIE F. GATES, PhD, RN, Professor and Director, Western Michigan University, Bronson School of Nursing, Kalamazoo, Michigan

MARY ENZMAN HAGEDORN, PhD, RN, CNS, CPNP, AHN-BC, Professor and Coordinator, DNP Program, Beth El College of Nursing and Health Sciences, University of Colorado at Colorado Springs, Colorado Springs, Colorado

VICKI D. JOHNSON, MSN, RN, CNAA, Clinical Assistant Professor of Nursing, College of Education and Human Services, School of Nursing, Cleveland State University, Cleveland, Ohio

MARGARET O'BRIEN KING, PhD, RNBC, AHNBC, Professor, Department of Nursing, College of Social Sciences, Health, and Education, Xavier University, Cincinnati, Ohio

CARLA MARIANO, EdD, RN, AHN-BC, FAAIM, Adjunct Associate Professor and former Coordinator, Advanced Adult Holistic Nurse Practitioner Program, New York University; and President, American Holistic Nurses Association, Flagstaff, Arizona

PAMELA J. POTTER, DNSc, ARNP, Senior Postdoctoral Fellow, Biobehavioral Nursing and Health Systems, University of Washington, Seattle, Washington

SHARON RADZYMINSKI, PhD, JD, RN, Graduate Program Director and Associate Professor, School of Nursing, College of Education and Human Services, Cleveland State University, Cleveland, Ohio

TERRY REED, RN, MS, HN-BC, Co-Founder and Co-Director, Beyond Ordinary Nursing, Certificate Program in Imagery, Foster City; and Guided Imagery Clinical Supervisor, Mills-Peninsula Health Services, Institute for Health and Healing, San Mateo, California

DIANE WIND WARDELL, PhD, RNC, Associate Professor, Department of Target Populations, School of Nursing, University of Texas Health Science Center–Houston, Houston, Texas

JANET WEBER, MSN, EdD, RN, Professor of Nursing, Coordinator of On-Campus RN to BSN Track, Department of Nursing, Southeast Missouri State University, Cape Girardeau, Missouri

ROTHLYN P. ZAHOUREK, PhD, APRN, BC, AHN-BC, Adjunct Clinical Faculty, University of Massachusetts, School of Nursing; and Private Practice, Holistic Psychotherapy, Amherst, Massachusetts

CONTENTS

Holistic nurses believe that the human being, composed of a mind, body and soul integrated into an inseparable whole that is greater than the sum of the parts, is in constant interaction with the universe and all that it contains. Health and well-being depend on attaining harmony in these relationships. Healing is the journey toward holism. Using presence, intent, unconditional acceptance, love, and compassion, holistic nurses can facilitate growth and healing and help their clients to find meaning in their life experiences, life purpose, and reason for being.

This article describes the *Holistic Nursing: Scope and Standards of Practice.* It defines holistic nursing, its five core values, and its practice standards. These include holistic philosophy, theory, and ethics; holistic caring process; holistic communication, therapeutic environment, and cultural diversity; holistic education and research; and holistic nurse self-care. Educational preparation for holistic nursing and settings in which holistic nurses practice are also explored.

Complementary and alternative healing modalities are increasing in popularity. Partially in response to client demand and partially because of a strong history in providing care encompassing the whole person, nurses have responded by incorporating selected alternative therapies within select professional services. There are questions, however, as to whether some or all of these modalities are within the boundaries of nursing practice. Because most professional practice acts are vague in relation to specific therapies, a model for legal analysis is presented.

Holistic assessment and care are inseparable from the nursing process. Holistic nursing practice informed by a philosophy of holism balancing art and science recognizes the interconnectedness of body, mind, and spirit. Holistic practice draws on knowledge, theories, expertise, intuition, and creativity. The purpose of this article is to place nursing in the context of holistic practice; to explicate the role of presence as an essential condition for holistic care; and to provide an example of the holistic caring process that incorporates theory, presence, and practice documented in the standard formats. A holistic approach to nursing integrates process and presence in the provision of care. Process alone is empty without presence. Presence alone is insufficient without the process.

This article explores more efficacious strategies for holistic nurses to promote healthy behavior choices in their clients. It presents an overview of self-determination theory (SDT) and describes research evidence that supports the application of SDT to promoting healthy behavior change in clients. When nurses act in ways that support clients' innate needs for autonomy, competence, and relatedness, clients may be more successful at internalizing self-regulation and more inclined to adopt and maintain lifelong behavioral changes. Some examples of nursing interventions to motivate behavior change are outlined in this article.

Research on touch therapies is still in the early stages of development. Studies of therapeutic touch, healing touch, and reiki are quite promising; however, at this point, they can only suggest that these healing modalities have efficacy in reducing anxiety; improving muscle relaxation; aiding in stress reduction, relaxation, and sense of well-being; promoting wound healing; and reducing pain. The multidimensional aspects of healing inherent in patient care continue to be expanded and facilitated by our understanding and application of energy therapies.

holistic nursing into curriculum and overcoming barriers to including holistic nursing in nursing education are discussed. Examples are provided through the experiences of two schools of nursing that successfully incorporated holistic nursing concepts.

Holistic nursing is a discipline focused on healing the whole person and dedicated to understanding and supporting the premise of holistic health of the patient and promoting healing in practitioners, patients, families, social groups, and communities. An explication of knowledge related to caring and healing in the human health experience and in holistic nursing is informed by the individual nurse's paradigmatic stance. Holistic nursing research is complex and focuses on healing, particularly healing of self, others, systems, and communities at large. This article discusses the competing paradigmatic perspectives, theoretic perspectives supporting holistic research, fundamental patterns of knowing and knowledge generation, a framework for holistic research, and the challenges of conducting holistic research. Recommendations for future research agenda are presented.

FORTHCOMING ISSUES

RECENT ISSUES

THE CLINICS ARE NOW AVAILABLE ONLINE!

Access your subscription at:
http://www.theclinics.com

NURSING
CLINICS
OF NORTH AMERICA

Nurs Clin N Am 42 (2007) xi–xiv

Preface

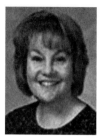

Noreen Frisch, PhD, RN, FAAN, APHN
Guest Editor

Evidence is all the rage in nursing these days, and the evidence-based practice (EBP) movement seems well-nigh unstoppable. Anyway, who would want to stop progress toward clinical care based on proven best practices? Many years ago, the nurse-scientist Dr. Norma Matheny reminded us how difficult it is to get any intervention/activity out of nursing practice once nurses are used to performing the activity. Nurses seem to be trapped in "we've always done it this way" kind of thinking, even when new knowledge shows a practice to be obsolete (or, worse, dangerous). Then, there is the equally daunting challenge of getting new ideas or procedures into clinical practice. This is often so slow that Rogers [1] wrote an entire book about how innovations "diffuse" into practice.

Even EBP itself diffuses slowly. Few practicing registered nurses (RNs) coming into my classes have a good understanding of evidence. That is unfortunate, because better understanding of the EBP movement would help us to use data wisely. I wonder, however, whether slow EBP diffusion is anywhere near as big a problem as is the troublingly limited understanding of some EBP "early adopters." Last spring, when discussing Watson's view of the essence of nursing as human caring, a student remarked that because she practiced on the basis of evidence only, she had no need to consider human connections—just the evidence and just the outcomes (measurable, of course), no more and no less. Well, she certainly had gotten some of the point of EBP, but had she missed the core of EBP, and of nursing itself?

So, I wondered: What have we done? As a holistic nurse, much of my reflection on practice has been guided by the philosophies and theories that

0029-6465/07/$ - see front matter © 2007 Published by Elsevier Inc.
doi:10.1016/j.cnur.2007.02.002   *nursing.theclinics.com*

permit us to view each person wholly and individually. Use of evidence requires sophistication in our discipline that we may not be imparting to our students—sophistication that we also may not be demanding of each other in our roles as research producers and research translators. Proper use of evidence requires an understanding of research methods, research designs, probability and statistics, ways of knowing, and levels of error. It also requires a solid understanding of the practical limits of evidence as we currently gather and interpret it. Applying evidence in practice is not a trivial process and has no "cookbook" schematic. As holistic nurses, we serve as teachers, guides, advocates, and supports to people who are dealing with significant health challenges and life situations. So, how does this occur in an era of EBP? I attempt to answer this question in the paragraphs that follow.

First, we must be certain our practitioners understand that we face many more clinical problems than we ever have clinical trials. Inevitably, much of what we do is based on good judgment without evidentiary proof. Second, we must be certain that our practitioners who read published research recognize that there are many more individual cases with variations than can be accounted for in our clinical trials. As Stephen Jay Gould famously wrote, after personal diagnosis of a rare cancer:

> Platonic heritage, with its emphasis in clear distinctions ... leads us to view statistical measures of central tendency wrongly ... as the hard "realities," and the variation that permits their calculation as a set of transient and imperfect measurements .... If the median is the reality and variation around the median just a device for its calculation, the "I will probably be dead in eight months" may pass as a reasonable interpretation. But all evolutionary biologists know that variation itself is nature's only irreducible essence. Variation is the hard reality .... Means and medians are the abstractions [2].

The randomized controlled clinical trial (RCT) is acknowledged as the "gold standard" of evidence. The controlled clinical trial provides the best data we have on how the average patient responds to the experimental interventions addressed in the study. As Gould reminds us, however, the average (mean or median) patient is an abstraction. Much of today's evidence is based on meta-analytic combinations of relatively small trials, often with moderately heterogeneous effect measures. If that heterogeneity is not carefully assessed (sometimes leading to the decision not to perform a meta-analysis), we may create "evidence" just as liable to error as the conclusion that Gould would live only 8 months (he died 20 highly productive years later of a different malignancy).

The goal of most RCTs is to reduce bias rather than to produce evidence applicable to clinical practice. Bias is most often reduced by enforcing strict exclusion criteria for participation in the trial. Few trials these days are "pragmatic" all-comer trials that can tell us whether a treatment is "effective" in real life. "Explanatory" RCTs establish what we call "efficacy"—an idea that

Gould would call "platonic." Participants are often selected only after a "run-in," during which their adherence is assessed, and they are often followed up more carefully than is possible in real life. Virtually all EBP is derived from studies of efficacy. What should matter to us is effectiveness: how well a treatment translates into practical real-life experience.

Real life also enters our thinking about trials in other ways. Our growing understanding of genetic polymorphisms reinforces the common sense idea (at the root of holistic nursing) that we are all different from one another. Single-subject studies offer effective ways to address these differences. The powerful N-of-1 trial technique is a quantitative variant of single-subject trials (as is the "within-person case crossover design," in which each individual acts as his or her own control). Neither study design is feasible in all circumstances, but both are useful in generating data that avoid abstraction.

Many people think that clinical trials determine "truth" independent of our prior knowledge or experience. To others, this concept is nonsensical. If evidence is not abstract truth, we need an entirely separate type of statistics, known as Bayesian reasoning, which has been developed to link statistical inference to individual likelihood. Used widely in genetics (Gould's field of endeavor), Bayesian statistics allow us to apply evidence to specific individual circumstances, something that is not possible with more traditional statistical results. Bayesian methods are not yet used in nursing studies, let alone in holistic nursing studies, although they should be adopted by both. These methods have begun to find their way into studies involving complementary and alternative therapies and also have articulate supporters in the internal medicine literature [3]. No one (especially Rogers) ever said that change comes quickly, but it seems that our need for evidence to use in practice should force us to take a serious look at why Bayesian methods based on individual inferences might serve our needs better than the more familiar frequentist model based on P values and null hypotheses.

Recently, Holmes and colleagues [4] presented a well-considered critique of what they called the "evidence-based dogma." These authors correctly point out that the EBP movement has served to reinforce a hierarchy of research designs that has prioritized frequentist quantitative methods over qualitative ones (and, I would add, over Bayesian or single-subject alternatives). Nursing, with its broad world view, seeks to understand the complexities of the lived experiences of those served, and it accepts ways of knowing that include esthetic, personal, and ethical knowledge as well as empiric knowledge. EBP in nursing requires consideration of evidence derived from a variety of points of view. Holistic nurses must ensure that evidence from a wide range of qualitative (and pragmatic or Bayesian) investigations inform practice decisions. We must not simply accept the hierarchy dictated by the current uncritical use of EBP. Just as Gould rescued himself by rejecting the tyranny of the median, so holistic nurses must rescue themselves and their clients from research methods enslaved to the mean and its distributions.

As we present the 11 articles that follow on philosophy/theory, scope of practice, modalities, education, care modalities, and research, we must do so in the context of EBP—the practical and pragmatic assumptions we bring to our care based on our experiences with real human beings, the data we obtain from research using a variety of investigative methods, and the practice decisions we make to assist our clients in their journey toward health.

It has been my privilege to compile and edit this issue. The work contained in it is a tribute to holistic care and a call for continuation of our need to build our body of knowledge in holism.

Noreen Frisch, PhD, RN, FAAN, APHN
School of Nursing, Cleveland State University
2121 Euclid Avenue
Cleveland, OH 44115, USA

E-mail address: n.frisch@csuohio.edu

References

[1] Rogers EM. The diffusion of innovations. 5th edition. New York: The Free Press; 2003.
[2] Gould SJ. The median isn't the message. Available at: http://edcallahan.com/web110/articles/gould.htm. Accessed December 2, 2006.
[3] Goodman SN. Toward evidence-based medical statistics. 2: the Bayes factor. Ann Intern Med 1999;130(12):1005–13.
[4] Holmes D, Perron A, O'Byrne P. Evidence, virulence, and the disappearance of nursing knowledge: a critique of the evidence-based dogma. Worldviews Evid Based Nurs 2006; 3(3):95–101.

NURSING
CLINICS
OF NORTH AMERICA

Nurs Clin N Am 42 (2007) 139–163

Philosophy and Theory of Holism

Helen L. Erickson, PhD, RN, AHN-BC, FAAN[a,b]

[a]*Holistic Adult Nursing, The University of Texas at Austin, Austin, TX, USA*
[b]*The American Holistic Nurses Certification Corporation, Cedar Park, TX, USA*

The concept that people are more than mind and body combined is as old as recorded time. Nevertheless, the term *holism* was not coined until the early twentieth century. Smuts, a South African statesman educated at Cambridge University and attracted to the work of the transcendentalists, concluded that there is a tendency in nature for the ordered grouping of units to create a whole [1]. He argued that this tendency occurs in the infinitesimal, such as the ordered structure of atoms that creates molecules, to the most complex forms of existence. Because his ideas were based in philosophy rather than science, his work, *Holism and Evolution* [2], was essentially overlooked for decades[1]. Today, many scientists credit the physicist Bohm [3,4] with the advancement of the concept of holism. Bohm's work with quantum mechanics reopened the door for Einstein's search for a unified energy field and universal consciousness—core concepts related to the understanding of holism today.

Conceptual derivations

The *term* holism, as defined by Smuts, was derived from the Greek word *holos*, which means whole. Nevertheless, the concept is probably rooted in the ancient Indian Vedic culture that existed thousands of years ago. Their Sanskrit language word, *sarvah*, meaning whole, intact, or uninjured, was used to describe [5] the nature of the human being as an integral part of the universe. More specifically, the word *sarvah* means that when the physical form of the human being is instilled with an omnipotent source of energy (or spirit) derived from the universe, it is whole, uninjured, and

E-mail address: helenerickson@mail.utexas.edu
[1] Few people realize that Smuts, based on his belief that systems are holistic (i.e. greater than the sum of the parts), facilitated the establishment of the League of Nations and wrote the Preamble for United Nations Charter.

doi:10.1016/j.cnur.2007.03.001

intact. The implication is that holism is the natural state of the human being; there should be interconnections within the human, between humans, and between humans and the universe. In the unnatural form, there is division among the components, the spirit is disconnected from the physical form, and the human is disconnected from the universe. This would cause "injury to the whole."

As cultures change, the meanings of concepts change too. For example, two words, *salvus* and *salus,* which came from the Roman culture, are thought to be derivatives of the Sanskrit word *sarvah.* The first, *salvus,* not only means uninjured but healthy and safe, whereas *salus* means good health. The Christian era verb save (derived from the Latin word *salvus*) means to deliver or rescue one's soul from peril. Similarly, a pre-Christian German word *halig* ("holy") means that which must be preserved whole or intact [5]. Thus, to extrapolate from past cultures, to be healthy is to have mind, body, and soul intact.

The current philosophy of holistic health care providers incorporates many of these definitions. Specifically, the human is composed of a mind, body, and soul integrated into a whole with inseparable parts. The whole is in dynamic interaction within itself, between and among other humans, and with the universe. When all parts are balanced and in harmony, maximum well-being exists. Well-being can exist in the presence or absence of physical ailment. Although health can be discussed in several ways—physical, social, emotional, cognitive, or spiritual health—to be truly healthy, one must experience a sense of well-being. An imbalance and disharmony within the human, human to human, and human to universe interfere with a person's well-being.

Practice derivations

Just as the concept of holism is not new, neither is the practice of holistic health care. For example, the ancient Vedic system for caring for the sick provides the philosophic basis for the modern-day Ayurveda holistic healing system. This model, recognized by the National Institutes of Health[2], is based on the belief that health problems occur when relationships among the person, the environment, and the universe are out of balance [6]. It assumes well-being is a natural state that occurs when people are facilitated to achieve balance in body, mind, and soul and are in harmony with the universe.

Nightingale [7] articulated similar beliefs when she stated that the nurse's role is to "... put the patient in the best condition for nature to act upon him." She stipulated that touch, kindness, and other comforting measures,

---

[2] This healing system was recognized by the National Institute of Health, CAM Division, as a Complementary and Alternative medical system.

provided within the context of a healing environment, are the crux of nursing. For 100 years, nurses built on these premises. Educators taught nurses how to manipulate the environment and use touch, massage, eye contact, soft voices, and other comforting measures so that people could get well. These nursing actions, known as the art of nursing, provided the underpinnings of professional nursing. Related assumptions were that the nurse's role was to help people get well, stay well, and have a peaceful death. Unfortunately, nurses often failed to recognize the importance of their care. As a result, as technology advanced, many discarded the age-old wisdom embedded in the art of nursing and turned to the values of other disciplines to articulate the essence of nursing.

Evolution of nursing philosophy

By the mid-1960s, several nurse leaders argued for systematic nursing based on the nurse-patient relationship [8] and for a science of nursing [9]. Using the reductionist model of medicine, in which the whole is the sum of the parts, graduate nursing programs were developed to help nurses learn how to become experts in a specific area of care. Most nurse experts were soon known by the part of the body, the type of problem, or the population they specialized in. Medical-surgical, psychiatric, obstetric, and pediatric nurses emerged. Standards of nursing were written to guide their practice [10]. Care of the human spirit and the soul was usually delegated to ministers, chaplains, and other religious leaders.

As nursing research expanded, emphasis shifted from the art of comforting and caring for holistic persons to the science of sickness and disease, often with an emphasis on a condition or medical diagnosis. Nurses became specialized in the care of people with specific types of organ or system conditions.

Division of thought

Not all nurses supported the movement toward specialization as defined in the 1960s and early 1970s. Although professional nurses supported the movement toward autonomy, some argued that nursing was a profession of caring [11,12] and should address the needs of the whole person rather than just the system or disease identified by a medical diagnosis.

By the late 1970s, two divisions of thought predominated nursing. The first group supported the philosophic paradigm embedded in the movement of the previous years. They believed that people were wholistic[3] (Fig. 1); in other words, psychosocial needs were important but the parts of the person

---

[3] Wholism is where the sum of the parts equals the whole. The implications are that the parts can be separated, studied, and treated.

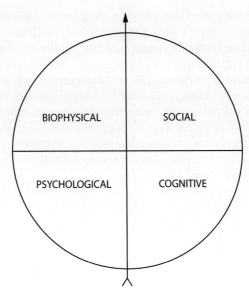

Fig. 1. Wholistic model. (*From* Erickson H, Tomlin E, Swain M. Modeling and role-modeling: a theory and paradigm for nursing. Engelwood Cliffs (NJ): Prentice-Hall, 1983. p. 46; with permission © 1983, EST Co.)

could be identified and treated in isolation to the rest of the person. Health was considered the absence, management, or control of a disease or condition. Well-being existed when the nurse or doctor determined that the person was healthy.

The second group argued for a holistic (Fig. 2) paradigm[4]. They believed that body, mind, and spirit were inextricably integrated and must be considered as a dynamic interactive unit with inseparable parts. Health was defined as a sense of well-being. Accordingly, people could die and still be healthy if they experienced comfort and peace in their mind and soul and were connected with loved ones. Under these circumstances, people were healthy when they perceived they were; they could experience a disease or condition but perceive themselves as healthy. Conversely, someone might have nothing more than a sense of "unease" and not be healthy. Well-being was purely subjective and determined by the client.

Although both groups agreed that the nurse's role was to address the needs of the person (not the disease), significant differences existed in how they operationalized their practice. Nurses who believed that people are wholistic often focused on the sickness or illness and perceived themselves as the experts in caring for the problem. They developed skills and expertise

---

[4] Holism is an inseparable integration of all components of the person, creating a whole that is greater than sum of the parts.

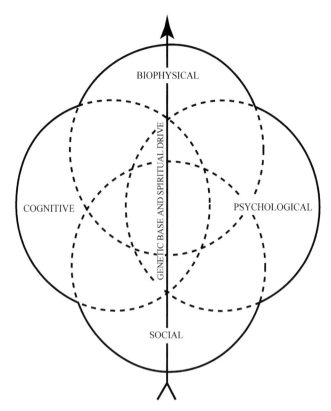

Fig. 2. Holistic model. (*From* Erickson H, Tomlin E, Swain M. Modeling and role-modeling: a theory and paradigm for nursing. Engelwood Cliffs (NJ): Prentice-Hall, 1983. p. 45; with permission © 1983, EST Co.)

often based on technology, pharmacology, pathophysiology, or psychopathology. Their nursing histories focused on objective data, such as system problems and conditions, and their care plans addressed objective data and paralleled the medical problem or diagnosis. The client's perspective, identified as subjective data, was usually considered insignificant or unrelated to the condition and frequently went unheeded. Sometimes, they recognized a compromise in their client's spiritual well-being but often viewed it as insignificant, unrelated to the problem of concern, or outside their expertise. People were often talked about as "the MI in bed 204" or "the gallbladder in Room 106." Nursing reports focused on medical orders, dressing changes, equipment management, what was wrong with the patients, and so forth.

At the same time, nurses who viewed people as holistic focused on individuals, families, or communities. They considered the medical problem, but it was not the focus of their care. Instead, they were concerned with their clients' perceptions and what they thought they needed to get well and experience a sense of interconnectedness. Believing that their clients were the experts, and therefore the primary source of information [13], they emphasized the importance of the caring and comforting aspects of professional activities. Their aim was to facilitate well-being in mind, body, and spirit. They knew that people who expressed hope and a will to live experienced their sickness or conditions differently from those who lacked these signs of spiritual well-being. Holistic nurses recognized that people were able to find meaning in their life experiences when they had hope, even when their physical life was threatened.

Many holistic nurses recognized the importance of stimulating the five senses as a way of facilitating balance and harmony in themselves and their clients. They used touch, music, massage, soft voice tones, quiet, and other nursing techniques and strategies that helped people to regain balance in mind, body, and spirit. They talked about the person, their perceived needs, and what nurses could do to help the person feel connected and comfortable. They recognized that the most important thing they could do for others is to actively listen to them and create a trusting working relationship with them.

Allegiance to two different philosophic paradigms impeded the profession's movement toward autonomy. Nursing leaders recognized the need to clarify professional nursing values and seek philosophic commonalities rather than differences; compromises were attempted. By 1980, the nursing's first social policy statement was published [14]. It stated that nurses focused on the "diagnosis and treatment of human responses to actual or potential health problems."

Emergence of holistic nursing

Although the social policy statement of the American Nurses Association (ANA) satisfied nurses who supported a wholistic model, many nurses felt disenfranchised. They continued to believe that the person, as an entity, cannot be broken down into parts or separated from the environment. They understood that people have organ systems but believed that nursing is concerned with the dynamic integration of all physical, social, emotional, cognitive, and spiritual components of the person. Furthermore, because people are inextricably linked to the environment, the well-being of one component of the system affects the well-being of others. This meant that nursing care is contextual; care of the holistic person mandates consideration of the context.

These nurses held firm to their belief that nursing of holistic persons is different from nursing of wholistic persons. Many dropped out of conventional health care systems and began searching for alternative ways to interact with clients. Some, building on their knowledge of the art of nursing, focused on the use of touch, aromas, music, yoga, meditation, exercise, communication strategies, and other modalities aimed at creating a healing environment and facilitating harmony and balance in the holistic being. Kinlein [15], the first nurse to go into private practice based on the holistic model, hung out her shingle as an independent nurse practitioner.

Concurrently, academic nurses who shared the holistic philosophy focused on articulating their beliefs; several conceptual models and theories emerged. Although many leaders provided guidance for nurses during this time, Rogers' [16] *Nursing: Science of Unitary Man* and Watson's [12] *Nursing: The Philosophy and Science of Caring* were particularly important in defining holistic nursing. These were followed by other works, such as Newman's [17] *Health as Expanding Consciousness*, Parse's [18] *Human Becoming*, and Erickson and colleagues' [13] *Modeling and Role-Modeling*. Others soon followed.

Central to each holistic nurse's philosophy were the beliefs that the whole is greater than the sum of the parts, the client's world view guides practitioners in understanding the whole, and the nurse is instrumental in helping people to heal and grow. Holistic nurses turned to one another for support. By the early 1980s, the American Holistic Nurses' Association (AHNA) [19] was organized under the leadership of Charlotte McGuire. Practitioners and academics merged together to label and articulate the essence of their philosophy. Within a few years holistic nursing core values were identified, standards of holistic nursing practice [20] were developed, continuing education programs were established to teach holistic nursing, and holistic nursing had emerged as a recognized national movement. Some concepts of holistic nursing were being incorporated into mainstream nursing, whereas others were not.

By 1997, the American Association of College of Nursing presented a position paper stating that baccalaureate nursing schools have the responsibility to provide education that emanates from nursing's core values, which include caring for the person, facilitating healing, and protecting the environment. The authors stated, "... in a nursing context, the distinction between disease and the illness experience lends understanding to the meaning of illness in a person's life. By itself, such meaning is a vital form of healing that can overcome the sense of alienation, loss of self, and loss of social integration that frequently accompany illness. This distinction is fundamental and unique to nursing" [21]. The two views in nursing were merging, but significant differences continued to exist. Holistic nurses, committed to their philosophy, identified the need for national certification. Under the direction and guidance of the AHNA, the American Holistic Nurses' Certification Corporation (AHNCC) was established [22]. By 2004, the AHNCC offered two examinations: the first to certify basic holistic nurses and the second to certify advanced holistic nurses. The respective acronyms are HN-BC and AHN-BC. A baccalaureate degree is the minimum educational level for the first, and a graduate degree is the minimal educational level for the second.

Today, the two philosophic paradigms continue to evolve, somewhat paralleling one another, often overlapping, and occasionally diverging along the lines of specific values and beliefs. For example, when the ANA social policy statement was revised in 2003, the values and assumptions that served as underpinnings for the statement were identified [23]. Although holistic nurses shared these values, many believed that they were not sufficiently articulated, and therefore left ambiguity in how they were applied. Furthermore, some beliefs held by holistic nurses diverge from those expressed by the ANA. A comparison of the two can be seen in Table 1.

Holism in the twenty-first century

Today, several disciplines, including physics, mathematics, science, philosophy, sociology, medicine, and nursing, support the view that the whole of an entity is more complex (or greater) than the sum of its parts. How this belief is applied varies with the discipline, however. For example, Greene [24], a quantum physicist, argues that all things in the universe are interconnected by energy particles, whereas theologists, such as Moore [25], address the interconnectedness and inseparability of man and God.

Health care providers, concerned with the macroscopic and microscopic views of life, defined their disciplines accordingly. For example, Pert [26], a research pharmacist, articulates mind-body connections by way of the science of psychoneuroimmunology, whereas physicians, such as Gerber [27], Dossey [28], and Chopra [29], draw from the basic and behavioral sciences, quantum physics, theology, ancient Ayurveda beliefs, and others to describe holistic medicine. Key concepts found in their work include vibrational energy, energy fields, life-energy systems, consciousness, cellular memory, psychoneuroimmunology, and healing.

Concurrently, nursing leaders, such as Dossey and colleagues [30], Rogers [31], Watson [32], Newman [33], Parse [34], Erickson and colleagues [13], and others [35], have similarly drawn from various disciplines, synthesized knowledge, and created conceptual frameworks and theories for holistic nursing. Central to each of these models is the integration of science and the art of nursing. Concepts common to holistic nursing are similar to those of holistic medicine. In addition, holistic nurses are concerned with caring and healing energy fields, presence, intent, unconditional acceptance, love, compassion, touch, and meaning in life. They are also concerned with self-care knowledge. These are described in more detail elsewhere in this article.

Practice implications

Holistic nurses believe that unity of mind, body, and spirit creates a system that is dynamically interconnected with the universe. These interconnections mandate that the whole cannot be broken down into parts; it must be

Table 1

Comparison of American Nurses Association assumptions and values with those of holistic nurses

American Nurses Association	Holistic nurses
Humans manifest an essential unity of mind, body, and spirit,	Humans manifest an essential unity of mind, body, and spirit. This entity is dynamic, in constant interaction with the environment (and universe), and cannot be separated or reduced to its parts.
Human experience is contextually and culturally defined.	Human experience is contextually and culturally defined, so nurses must attempt to understand their clients' view of their world.
Health and illness are human experiences. The presence of illness does not preclude health, nor does optimal health preclude illness.	Health and illness are human experiences. Nurses help people to discover meaning in these experiences.
The relationship between nurse and patient occurs within the context of values and beliefs of the patient and the nurse.	Same
Public policy and the health care delivery system influence the health and well-being of society and professional nursing.	Same
	Therapeutic nursing interventions require that the nurse and client merge as a holistic unit. This happens during the caring process.
	Nurses facilitate the caring process by creating a nurturing environment.
	Because of the interconnectedness of nurse and client, holistic nurses must integrate self-care into their own lives.
	The focus of nursing is to promote well-being, the context is the caring process, and the goals are facilitating growth and development and healing (as needed).
	People have self-care knowledge; it is the primary source of information.
	Holistic nurses can use alternative and complementary nursing strategies and modalities to facilitate a caring environment and holistic healing.

considered as a dynamic interactive entity that exists within a context. A person cannot be reduced to an entity composed of a set of systems, such as the neurologic, cardiac, renal, or hepatic system. People cannot be defined as members of a population, such as psychiatric or medical-surgical patients, or as members of a group, such as a mother, father, friend, nurse, or client. They must be thought of as an entity in which the whole is greater than the sum of its parts, interconnected with other people directly and indirectly by way of the universe. Many holistic nurses turn to quantum physics to help them understand these beliefs.

Holism and energy fields

Einstein [36] stated, "A human being is a part of the whole, called by us the Universe, a part limited in time and space. He experiences himself, his thoughts and feelings as something separated from the rest—a kind of optical delusion of his consciousness." Key to Einstein's statement is that all things are connected to one another, from the smallest component in the universe to the largest. According to Gribbin [37], these connections occur by way of subatomic particles that can change unceasingly into each other; they can manifest as mass or energy. Brekke and Schultz [38] simplify this by stating:

> The theory of quantum physics holds that protons and neutrons are each made up of very small particles called quarks. They are held together by even smaller particles called gluons, which collect together to make glueballs! They are so small we cannot observe them directly—they are subatomic particles .... These subatomic particles are very resourceful and can manifest as a particle or a wave.

Suffice it to say that these tiny subatomic particles work together to create currents of energy. They also work with gravity to create electromagnetic energy fields [38]. Although the human body seems to be solid matter, it is transformed energy. The cells of the body are continuously interacting with one another, providing information about the person as a whole, creating energy fields. The energy fields of the body are continuously interacting with one another and with those of the environment. There is a continuous exchange of information by way of energy flow. When taken as a whole, a repository of knowledge is created[5], a repository of knowledge that some call universal consciousness. Holistic nurses believe that people can tap into this repository of knowledge to help them grow and become.

Mind-body-soul connections

Pert [39], one of the early psychoneuroimmunology scientists connecting mind and body by way of chemical molecules, says that "energy is the free flow of information," cell to cell. To quote:

> What is this energy that is referred to by so many ... who associate it with the release of emotion and the restoration of health?... It is my belief that this mysterious energy is actually the free flow of information carried by the biochemicals of emotion, the neuropeptides and their receptors.

Pert's work on how the cells of the body communicate with one another, within an organ and between organs, is known as the science of psychoneuroimmunology [40]. It has provided holistic practitioners with a much deeper understanding of concepts, such as "cellular memory," "stored memories,"

---

[5] This is also known as Consciousness or Collective Consciousness. See Dossey, Keegan and Guzzetta [30] and Erickson [41] for more information.

and "state-dependent memories" [41], which seem to be information stored in the cells of the body by way of chemicals—memories waiting for triggers to stimulate their retrieval.

Holistic nurses believe that the science of psychoneuroimmunology helps them to understand better how the systems of the mind-body interact. It provides information about linkages between the brain, peripheral nervous system, and other systems of the body, including the immune system. This type of information is crucial in the understanding of the linkages between feelings, thoughts, and biophysical responses.

Nurses also believe that it is important to understand metabolic, bioelectrical, and chemical energy fields. For example, it is important for nurses to understand the creb cycle, electromagnetic conductive system of the heart, and transmission of messages from cell to cell by way of chemicals and hormones [42]. This knowledge is insufficient, however; it does not address two key beliefs of holistic nurses (that the soul is an integral part of the holistic person and that the person is inextricably connected to the universe). This type of knowledge requires moving beyond what can be seen in the laboratory. It requires a basic belief in and understanding of subtle energy that comes from a unified field of energy.

Einstein first proposed that there is a unified field of energy from which all energy emerges. Greene [24] drew from quantum physics in an attempt to explain how this works. His discussion of string theories I and II is compelling and offers some evidence that subtle energy probably exists. The presence of subtle energy remains substantially unproven, however. Nevertheless, most holistic nurses, many holistic physicians, and others believe that it does exist and that it is probably what many call the spiritual energy of the human being. It is what people tap into when they draw from universal energy or life force energy.

The concept of universal energy has been accepted in many cultures for centuries. Nevertheless, most traditional physicians and many wholistic nurses do not accept the idea of subtle energy, although they use energy-related procedures in everyday practice. Gerber [27], for example, states that Western medicine has come to recognize the human energy fields and, in fact, to use them to understand better the functioning of the human body through the use of sonograms, radiographs, and MRI, for example. Still, traditional Western medicine fails to recognize subtle energy. He states, "These other energy systems (ie, subtle energy) are the important life-energy and spiritual-energy systems of the multidimensional human being" [27].

Gerber is not alone in his beliefs. Many advocates of the concept of holistic human beings believe that subtle energy is an expression of the soul, our link to a higher power. Pert [26], for example, stated:

> In a very real sense, our Soul, our 'true self,' expresses itself through a physical body that is subtly influenced and molded by these various spiritual bodies. Each of our spiritual bodies is formed from vibrating life-energy

fields of progressively higher and finer levels of energy and matter ... invisible to the naked eye .... It provides a unique form of energetic information to the cells of the body that help guide human growth and development.

Subtle energy fields in and around the human body are described by holistic practitioners as the human energy system [38]. This system consists of meridians, chakras, and the auric (energy) field. The meridians are described as pathways along which energy flows. Chakras are sites (known as a vortex) where meridians intersect, creating a continuous spinning of energy[6]. When chakras get blocked, energy flow is diminished. The aura is the energy field created within and around the human body. These energy fields are known as auric fields. Energy-focused practitioners assess the auric field to determine balance (or imbalance) within the human energy system. Based on their findings, they facilitate energy flow through the chakras and meridians. It is believed that health and well-being depend on the continuous flow of energy within the body, between people, and among people and other components of the universe.

Rogers' [43] nursing theory, *Nursing: A Science of Unitarian Human Beings*, was the first to provide guidelines for nurses who viewed people within this context. Kunz and Kreiger [44] extrapolated from Rogers' work to develop the modality commonly known as Therapeutic Touch. Mentgen [45] followed with Healing Touch [46], a comprehensive model that incorporates energy theory with other principles that help to balance the physical, mental, emotional, and spiritual aspects of the person. Other modalities, including Reiki, yoga, meditation, and tai chi, [47] have also been built on energy therapies.

Caring field

Watson [12], whose seminal work maintains that caring is central to nursing, incorporated energy concepts into her philosophy [32] to describe the "caring field." She stated that a caring field occurs when the nurse and client connect on an energetic level and went on to say that a caring field creates new possibilities for the well-being of both participants. Other nurse theorists have also incorporated the concept of interconnectedness between nurse and client, arguing that the relationship has the potential to affect their well-being. For example, according to Rogers [16], whose entire nursing theory is energy based, "Professional practice in nursing seeks to promote symphonic interaction between human and environmental fields, to strengthen integrity of the human field, and to direct and redirect patterning of the human and environmental fields for realization of maximum health potential." Newman [33], whose work is grounded in Rogers' model, stated that the nurse's role is "... to help clients get in touch with the meaning of their lives by identification of their patterns of relating ...." She goes on to say, "Intervention is a form of nonintervention whereby the nurse's *presence* assists clients to recognize

---

[6] If one could visualize this, it might look like a spinning pinwheel.

their own patterns of interacting with the environment" [33]. Both authors allude to the nature of the caring field as the process or the outcome.

Erickson and colleagues [13], authors of the modeling and role-modeling nursing model, also address the interconnectedness between nurse and client and its potential effect on clients. They state, "Nursing is ... the interactive, interpersonal process that nurtures strengths to enable development, release, and channeling of resources for coping with one's circumstances and environment." They go on to state that nursing is based on five key principles; the first is "The nursing process requires that a trusting and functional relationship exist between nurse and client" [13]. They state that people have an inherent need to be connected while maintaining a sense of independence; that is, people need to have a "... deep sense of both the 'I' and the 'we' states of being and to perceive freedom and acceptance in both states" [13]. They call this affiliated-individuation. Later, Brekke and Schultz [38] add to this by stating:

> The auric field (a component of the human energy system) can be used to explain affiliated-individuation at the energetic level. Because we are in constant interaction with the environment, it is difficult to identify a specific point where a person's auric field ends and the 'Universe' starts. However, we can perceive the boundaries of the auric field.

They offer a way to visualize the caring field as the interacting auras of two people (Fig. 3). They illustrate the intersection of the two energy fields, creating a field between the two people that is great enough to affect their auric boundaries. They also illustrate the human's need for individuation by way of energy that is not completely overlapping with that of another. The implications are that people within the caring field experience a closeness and interconnectedness by means of which they feel safe and cared about.

For comparison, Brekke and Schultz [38] also offer a visual representation of two people, near one another, whose energy fields are not synchronized. The result is lack of connection or an absence of a caring field (Fig. 4). Although there is a field of interaction, they have not created a caring field. The implications in this situation are that the people involved feel isolated and uncertain of the one another; they are unable to draw healing energy— energy needed to get well, grow, and develop—from the relationship.

McKivergin and Daubenmire [48] addressed this when they stated:

> The nurse has a profound effect on the patient and we need to assume responsibility for awareness of the effect. As we become increasingly aware of this oneness, this interconnectedness, we can view the nurse-patient encounter as a dynamic, open, ever-changing energy system. There is a continuous multilevel exchange of energy between nurse and client.

Dossey [49] said that nurses affect the caring field through their intentions, feelings, and thought. When nurses intend to facilitate movement toward holism in their clients, the caring field can become a healing field.

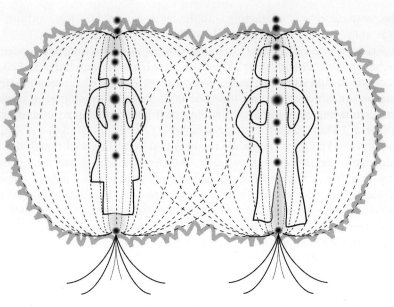

Fig. 3. Energy fields and joint aura of two people positively interacting with one another. (*From* Brekke M, Schultz E. Energy Theories. In: Erickson H, editor. Modeling and role-modeling: a view from the client's world. Cedar Park (TX): Unicorns Unlimited Book Publishers; 2006. p. 59; with permission.)

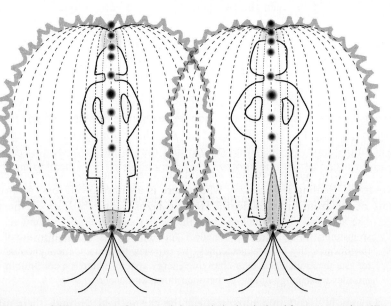

Fig. 4. Energy fields and auras of two people in proximity but isolated from one another. (*From* Brekke M, Schultz E. Energy Theories. In: Erickson H, editor. Modeling and role-modeling: a view from the client's world. Cedar Park (TX): Unicorns Unlimited Book Publishers; 2006. p. 60; with permission.)

Healing field

Kinney [50] argues that healing starts when an energy field is created between two people. Kaliscchuk and Davies [51] define healing as the "journeying toward wholism." It occurs as people move toward holism. The outcome is a healthy integrated balance between mind, body, and soul that produces a harmony within the human being. McTaggart [52] states that people might facilitate healing (through the healing field) in two different ways. First, a person may act as an energy conduit allowing the recipient's energy field to realign, and second, the healing energy field may be "... a collective memory of healing spirit." Healing spirit, or subtle healing energy, is believed to come from the universe and is described as Mana, Prana, Ki, Chi, Chee, Ci, Rauch, and Barrake depending on the culture. It is believed to be drawn from the life force, life energy, or God [38].

Holistic nurses believe that people have an inherent spiritual drive, a need to have mind, body, and soul integrated. As shown in Fig. 1, the human's spiritual drive draws from the universe and gives to the universe [53]. As universal energy is drawn into the physical being, it is transformed, used, and redistributed through multiple methods (including the chakras and meridians). This is the healing process, and nurses can facilitate the healing process by creating a healing field.

Although it may seem that a caring field and a healing field are the same, there are some differences. A caring field occurs when there is intent to synchronize energy fields and facilitate growth in both participants. The nurse's goal is to establish perceptions of safety and to enhance the overall comfort and well-being of both participants. A healing field is an extension of a caring field. Both require that the nurse aim to synchronize the two independent energy fields and have the intent to facilitate growth by way of balancing the energy fields of the other member of the dyad. The aim is to create a sense of safety and comfort. In comparison, the nurse entering the healing field also has the intent to help the other person build resources needed to reorganize the mind-body-soul configuration and create holistic well-being. The aim is not only to create a sense of safety and comfort but to help people release unhealthy cellular "memories," replace them with healthy growth-related chemicals, and increase developmental strengths. Healing is necessary when there is an unresolved loss, a natural part of life from birth to death. Healing helps people to "bridge the gap between loss and Self-discovery" [54].

Sometimes nurses enter the caring field with intent to facilitate growth and, unknown to themselves, enter the healing field. This is because humans have a natural propensity to grow, develop, and heal when they are safely connected with another human being while simultaneously feeling that they have permission to be individuated. In other words, they have a healthy balance in affiliated-individuation [13,55]. The caring and healing processes are based on reciprocal relations between the two members of the partnership. Language, feelings, attitudes, and behaviors of one person influence those of the other. This is why it is important for nurses to know themselves well and to use self-care strategies to help themselves become integrated—mind, body, and soul [53,56,57].

Interestingly, growth and healing sometimes continue long after the initial encounter. This may be because nurses who use intent may stay energetically connected through time and space. In addition, because people have an inherent natural tendency to heal given the opportunity, once the healing process is initiated, it continues through time and space [58]. Watson [59] would call this "transpersonal caring," and Erickson [58] calls it the "long arm effect." Nurses have the potential to have an impact on their clients long after they have physically separated from them.

Presence

Parse [60], another mentee of Rogers, adds to the understanding of the caring-healing energy field by introducing the concept of presence. She states:

> The nurse is in true presence with the individual (or family) as the individual (or family) uncovers the personal meaning of the situation and makes choices to move forward in the now moment with cherished hopes and dreams. The focus is on the meaning of the lived experience for the person (or the family) unfolding *there with* the presence of the nurse ....

The concept of presence, basic in holistic nursing, and a prerequisite for creating a caring-healing field is not new to nursing. Nightingale [7] alluded to presence in her lengthy discussion of the nurse as observer and the one who provides comforting care, stating that nursing observations are "... not for the sake of piling up miscellaneous information or curious facts, but for the sake of saving life and increasing health and comfort." Throughout her work, she emphasized the need for the nurse to be able to "... distinguish between the idiosyncrasies of patients" [7], recognize changes in client well-being, and provide comfort so that nature can take its course—to relieve pain and suffering and heal the sick. Although never stated, Nightingale's *Notes on Nursing* imply that good observational skills, a necessary nursing activity, depend on the nurse being present with the client.

Paterson and Zderad [61] defined presence as being open and giving of oneself to the relationship between nurse and client. Many others have also described presence, including some nurse theorists. For example, according to Watson [12,62], it is a connection that occurs between nurse and client, and Parse [63] described it as attentiveness.

The modeling and role-modeling theory [53] also incorporates the concept of a caring presence. As stated, "Our goal is to be Present, to have Presence, so we can help our clients help themselves. We do this first by centering ourselves; this organizes our energy. Next, we focus our intent, which helps us direct our energy and draw from the Universe. Finally, we open ourselves to our client, so our energy fields can merge" [53]. The implication is that presence requires active participation on the nurse's part (centering [of self], focused intent on the client, and opening of their energy fields to facilitate synchronization of the two fields).

Covington [64] compiled the work of more than 70 authors and presented a concept analysis of presence. She concluded that it is a way of being, being with, and relating with others. She concluded that "Caring Presence is an interpersonal, intersubjective human experience of connection within a nurse-patient relationship that makes it safe for sharing oneself with another" [64].

Intentionality

Intentionality, a concept based on energy theory and basic to holistic nursing, is also prerequisite for creating a caring field and a healing field. Intention, based on feelings and thoughts, affects the direction of energy flow. Simply stated, energy follows intent. When the nurse intends to facilitate growth and development in another person, the nurse's energy field synchronizes with the client's, making it possible for them to create a holistic energy field between them. When people say such things as, "I'm so sorry about your loss. I'll send you some energy and hope that it helps you," and they mean what they are saying, they are using intent. Holistic nurses believe that intent, directed purposefully, can have a powerful impact on others. Some research [42] has shown that intentionality, even when the two participants are separated by distance, can have a positive effect on the well-being of the recipient of the intent. Some, such as Chopra [65], Dossey [49], and Gerber [27], argue that our intent to help people creates a healing field, irrespective of time and space. Waters and Daubenmire [66] stated that "the essence of nursing lies in creating a healing environment and in engaging the patient's consciousness in the healing process." They went on to say that intentionality is key to creating a healing environment.

If energy follows intent, consider what happens when nurses enter the space of another with the intent of checking the equipment or other inanimate objects in the room. Because energy follows intent, their energy is directed toward that object. Their touch might be perceived as aggressive and discomforting. Humans in the room experience the lack of "connection" with the nurse; they often feel unimportant, isolated, alone, and unsafe. Sometimes, they perceive that they have been assaulted rather than comforted.

In comparison, when humans enter the space of another with the intent to care for the person while managing the equipment, energetic connections are created. A caring-healing field results. Sometimes, with as little as a smile, eye contact, gentle touch, or quiet words of reassurance, clients experience a sense of safety and comfort—they are put in the best possible condition to heal.

Unconditional acceptance

Presence and intentionality are prerequisites for creating a caring-healing energy field; so is unconditional acceptance. When discussing unconditional acceptance, the key question is what is being unconditionally accepted? When holistic nurses say they believe in unconditional acceptance, they mean that they recognize and accept the human being as a sacred entity of the universe—a human being who has an inherent need to grow and become fully integrated mind, body, and soul. Within this context, holistic nurses also recognize the inherent need for all humans to feel safe, to be loved and respected, to have a sense of self-worth, and to find meaning in their lives. This does not mean that holistic nurses accept or approve of behaviors and attitudes that are hurtful to the individual or others. It simply means that holistic nurses value the need of all people to be respected and viewed as worthy human beings, even when they participate in antisocial behaviors. When someone experiences unconditional acceptance, they begin to experience "… a sense of worth and dignity, trust in the provider, discovery that one's Self is what is important, the ability to listen to one's Inner Voice, and the initiation of a natural, self-healing process" [67]. Caring is what we do as nurses, interfacing heart-to-heart. It is the essence of nurturing. "Healing is what we aim to facilitate in our clients who seek help with becoming more fully holistic" [58]. To create a healing field, nurses must have the intent to facilitate growth and development and to facilitate people to heal. Although unconditional acceptance of the human's need for safety, respect, self-worth, and dignity is a prerequisite for creating a caring field, nurses who wish to extend the caring field into a healing field must also unconditionally accept the human without expectations of who he or she becomes. Unconditional acceptance is the basis for love and loving.

Love

To love, within the context of holistic nursing, is to show grace and charity toward another human being and to feel compassion, the type of compassion shown to humanity by God. Gerber [68] argues that learning to love is perhaps the most difficult thing there is to learn as a human being. He goes on to say that without love, existence can be meaningless and that we not only need to learn to love those around us but ourselves.

Newman [17] talks about love, stating that it is "… the substrate for all emotion. It manifests itself in different forms depending on the person's ability to *let go* and let love be." She goes on to say that "… love is there, people just don't know how to let it out" [17]. Later, she draws from Moss [69,70] to say that unconditional love is the embracing of all experience, a state of awareness without judgment.

Kinney [50], drawing from several sources, including the HeartMath Institute [71], concluded that the heart has the strongest electromagnetic field in the body. Energetically, it is a cyclic reciprocal relation between the soul and spirit. Unconditional love, a precursor to unconditional acceptance, comes from being connected with the universe. When people connect heart-to-heart, it is possible for them to go to the next step and connect spirit-to-spirit. This is the essence of love.

Compassion

What then is the difference between the concepts of love and compassion? Keegan and Dossey [72] describe compassion as "... a way of being that can be enhanced as we develop our inner awareness of our various relationships with self and other." They go on to say that this involves all things in the "living and non-living world." Others, such as Steere [73], relate compassion to nurturing and being kind. He draws an analogy with "... kindly sheep herders gathering the lambs in their arms, giving careful attention to the young, the lame, or the vulnerable." Perhaps this is comparable to Nightingale's discussion of the nurse's role as a monitor, observer, and comforter.

Compassion and love are closely linked, although there seems to be a major difference: the essence of unconditional love is being connected spiritually within oneself and with the spirit of others. It is a way of experiencing self and others without judgments or values. Compassion entails loving but includes the component of being aware of the human condition and its vulnerability. Compassion is an understanding of and acceptance of the human condition and its vulnerabilities. Holistic nurses seek unconditional love and strive to develop compassion.

Finding meaning

Life is a journey, and there is a purpose for the journey [74]. It is not just a happenstance series of events. Although the pathways people take are influenced by their actions and decisions, there is a reason for being that is related to the holistic self. Each journey is filled with human experiences; some are wonderful, and some are not. Nevertheless, each experience can contribute to fulfillment of one's purpose in life.

Holistic nurses aim to help people find meaning in their life experiences so that they can continue to grow and to become [75], or, as Newman [70] would say, to expand their consciousness. This is not a matter of understanding disease processes; it is a matter of discovering what a disease, condition, or event can teach us about our own life purpose and our reason for being [74]. When people are unable to find meaning in their experiences, they often suffer; they are disconnected body and soul.

One author said, "Meaningless suffering can lead to spiritual disintegration. Finding meaning in the experience can be an attenuator of how the event is experienced" [76]. Clayton [77] calls these meaningless experiences invisible wounds. She describes the effect they have on the overall well-being of people as they continue on their journey, sometimes stumbling because it is hard to find their way. She goes on to describe the role of the nurse in helping people to discover meaning in their life experiences and how this relieves suffering and helps people to grow.

Finding meaning in life circumstances can be an "ah-ha" experience, in which the light bulb suddenly seems to come on, an epiphany occurs, and the individual views life differently. Conversely, it can be a gradual seeping into one's awareness and a slow but certain change in perspective on life.

Finding meaning helps people to become more holistic and more integrated mind, body, and soul. Sometimes, it happens because of something a holistic nurse has purposefully done to help clients become better integrated; sometimes it happens because the natural tendency of the human being is to heal. When humans feel safe, loved, and connected, healing begins to happen; the meaning of life experiences becomes a part of their conscious understanding; and they grow and become more fully who they were meant to be.

Self-care knowledge

People have an inherent ability to grow and become the most that they can be, but they sometimes need help discovering what they are not consciously aware of but already know at some level in their being. This is because all humans have self-care knowledge [13], an inner voice or inner wisdom [78]. People know what has caused their sickness, lessened their effectiveness, and interfered with their growth. They also know what is going to help them maximize their effectiveness and promote their growth. This type of knowledge cannot be categorized as cognitive, psychosocial, or physical information because it is knowledge about their life purpose and reason for being. People are holistic; they are in human form because they need human experiences to help them do their soul-work [74]. They need nurses to nurture them and help them with this work.

Holistic nurses understand that their clients' self-care knowledge is the primary source of information. It is where nursing starts; it is the focus of caring. Although other sources of information, such as families and friends (ie, the secondary source of information), and sometimes medical information (ie, tertiary source of information), are also important, the human's self-care knowledge is primary. Take, for example, the client who has been admitted to the hospital with a diagnosis of a myocardial infarct. The nurse observes that this person seems agitated and has trouble breathing; however, when asked to describe the situation and what is needed, the client states that it is imperative that he speak with his wife immediately. Holistic nurses would understand that speaking with the wife has significance that is not obvious but must be addressed while simultaneously providing measures that relieve the strain on the cardiac system.

Because people are holistic, mind-body-spirit relations exist. When one part of the system is out of balance, it affects the entire system. Similarly, when self-care needs are addressed, even when they do not seem to have anything to do with the physical problem, the entire system is able to move toward a more balanced state. This affects the biochemistry of the body as well as all other aspects of the person. Most nurses have had the experience of a patient who seems to improve suddenly even though the nurse has not done anything other than listen or respond to some seemingly nonimportant request. This is because the nurse has addressed the client's needs by respecting and responding to his or her self-care knowledge. They nurture and facilitate mobilization and building of resources needed to acquire a balance and harmony among the multiple components of the whole being.

Nurses often have difficulty with this concept. Sometimes, they say that the person can die while holistic nurses are taking care of his or her emotional needs. Holistic nurses would not agree. They believe that what a person feels and thinks has a profound effect on his or her physical well-being and is often the root of the physical problem. Furthermore, because people know what is going to help them, unless their needs are addressed, their physical problem can get worse. Finally, they believe that what happens to an individual is affected by the nurse's intent, because energy follows intent. When the intent is to comfort the person and create a safe environment for healing to occur, a caring-healing field is created, reversing cascades of harmful neurotransmitters [42] and helping the individual to mobilize resources needed to contend with the physical assault. These nurses know it is important to make eye contact, speak in quiet voice tones, touch gently, and address the individual's need to connect with his wife, while concurrently administering oxygen and addressing other physical needs. Caring for the person rather than the disease is not difficult; it just requires that the nurse recognize self-care knowledge as primary information and act accordingly. In doing so, nurses help people to live their lives fully and, when it is time, to die peacefully.

Summary

Historically, medicine addressed the treatment of sickness and diseases, whereas nurses focused on the person. Physicians used the basic sciences to help them understand how to treat the focus of their interest, whereas nurses used the art of nursing to comfort their patients and help to restore balance within the person and between the person and the environment. The nurse's goal was to create a healing environment so that nature could take its natural course and people could get well or die peacefully.

Today, holistic nurses integrate the art and science of nursing to create a caring-healing environment for the same reason. They also use research findings from other disciplines, such as the science of psychoneuroimmunology, which describes relations between the mind and body, and energy theories, which describe relationships between and among people and the universe. They believe that the human being—composed of a mind, body, and soul integrated into a dynamically interactive inseparable whole—is in constant interaction with the universe and all that it contains. Health and well-being depend on attaining harmony in these relationships.

Holistic nurses argue that people know what causes imbalance and disharmony and what they need to acquire a sense of well-being; this type of "knowing" is called self-care knowledge. Caring is what nurses do, interfacing heart-to-heart, as they address their client's self-care knowledge. Their aim is to promote healing; their goal is to facilitate health and well-being, which can exist in the presence or absence of physical ailment. They synchronize their own energy fields with their client's to create caring-healing environments. When they do this, they use gentle comforting touch, presence, intent, unconditional acceptance, love, and compassion.

Presence is a state of opening oneself to the needs of another, without expectations or distractions. Presence does not require doing something; instead, it is a way of being or being with someone. It is a way of relating with another human being when the focus is on the well-being of the other. Holistic nurses also use intentionality, the concentrated focus of energy. Intentionality occurs when nurses deliberately center their attention on an object or person. Holistic nurses use intentionality to focus their energy and synchronize energy fields so that they can create a caring-healing environment.

Unconditional acceptance of the human as a being of the universe without expectations of who he or she becomes is an essential prerequisite for facilitating healing. When holistic nurses unconditionally accept the essence of another human being, they recognize the inherent need of all people to be valued and to have self-worth and self-dignity. Unconditional acceptance of the essence of another human being is the basis for love and loving. To love is to show compassion for the human, without judgment or values. Compassion not only includes love but is an understanding of human nature, the human condition, and its vulnerabilities.

Holistic nurses recognize that birth, death, and all experiences in between are a part of the human journey. They aim to help people become more fully holistic—more fully integrated mind, body, and spirit—as they travel their pathways. As healing occurs, people find meaning in their unique life experiences. They become more fully aware of their potential and their life purpose. When this happens, people are able to live life more fully, transcend the physical plane more peacefully, and grasp the full meaning of their reason for being, their soul-work.

Acknowledgments

Editorial assistance was provided by Geeta Erickson, MA, and graphics by Lance M. Erickson, MA.

References

[1] Lawrence C, Weisz GT. Greater than the parts: holism in biomedicine, 1920–1950. New York: Oxford University Press; 1998. p. 2–5.
[2] Smuts J. Holism and evolution. New York: MacMillian Company; 1926.
[3] Bohm D. Wholeness and the implicate order. London: Routledge; 1980.
[4] Bohm D, Hiley BJ. The undivided universe. New York: Routledge; 1993.

[5] Entomology dictionary. Available at: http://www.etymonline.com. Accessed September 30, 2006.

[6] Chopra A, Doiphode V. Ayurvedic medicine—core-concept, therapeutic principles, and current relevance. Med Clin North Am 2002;86(1):75–88.

[7] Nightingale F. Notes on nursing: what it is and what it is not. New York: Dover Publications, Inc.; 1969. p. 133, 117–25.

[8] Orlando I. The dynamic nurse-patient relationship. New York: G.P. Putnam's Sons; 1961.

[9] Fawcett J. The relationship between theory and research: a double helix. ANS Adv Nurs Sci 1978;1(1):49–62.

[10] American Nurse's Association. Standards of clinical nursing practice. Washington, DC: ANA Publ; 1974.

[11] Abdellah F. Patient-centered approaches to nursing. New York: Macmillan; 1963.

[12] Watson J. Nursing: the philosophy and science of caring. Boston: Little Brown; 1979. p. 8–9.

[13] Erickson H, Tomlin E, Swain M. Modeling and role-modeling: a theory and paradigm for nursing. Engelwood Cliffs (NJ): Prentice-Hall; 1983. p. 116–48, 170–1.

[14] American Nurses' Association. Nursing: a social policy statement. Washington, DC: ANA Publ; 1980.

[15] Kinlein L. Independent nursing practice with clients. Philadelphia: J.B. Lippincott Company; 1977.

[16] Rogers M. An introduction to the theoretical basis of nursing. Philadelphia: F.A. Davis; 1970. p. 122.

[17] Newman M. Health as expanding consciousness. St Louis (MO): Mosby; 1986. p. 102.

[18] Parse R. Man-living-health: a theory of nursing. New York: Wiley; 1981.

[19] Available at: www.AHNA.org. Accessed October 20, 2006.

[20] American Holistic Nurses Association. Standards of holistic nursing practice. Flagstaff (AZ): AHNA Publications; 1992.

[21] American Association of Colleges of Nursing. AACN position statement, a vision of baccalaureate and graduate nursing education: the next decade. Available at: http://www.aacn.nche.edu/Publications/positions/vision.htm. Accessed October 16, 2006.

[22] Available at: http://ahncc.org/pages/1/index.htm. Accessed October 16, 2006.

[23] American Nurse's Association. Nursing's social policy statement American Nurses Association. Washington, DC: ANA Publications; 2003. p. 3.

[24] Greene B. The elegant universe. New York: Delta; 2003.

[25] Moore T. Care of the soul: a guide for cultivating depth and sacredness in everyday life. New York: HarperPerennial; 1992.

[26] Pert C. Molecules of emotion: the science behind mind-body medicine. New York: Scribner; 2003. p. 23.

[27] Gerber R. A practical guide to vibrational medicine: energy healing and spiritual transformation. New York: Quill, HarperCollins Publishers; 2001. p. 16.

[28] Dossey L. But is it energy? Reflections on consciousness, healing and the new paradigm. Subtle energies and energy medicine; 2002;3(3).

[29] Chopra D. Quantum healing: exploring the frontiers of mind-body medicine. 2nd edition. New York: Bantam; 1990.

[30] Dossey B, Keegan L, Guzetta C. Holistic nursing: a handbook for practice. 4th edition. Boston: Jones and Bartlett Publishers; 2005.

[31] Rogers M. Nursing: a science of unitary man. In: Reihl JP, Roy C, editors. Conceptual models for nursing practice. 2nd edition. New York: Appleton-Century-Crofts; 1980. p. 329–37.

[32] Watson J. Postmodern nursing and beyond. Edinburgh (UK): Churchill Livingstone; 1999.

[33] Newman M. Health as expanding consciousness. 2nd edition. New York: NLN Press; 1994. p. 499.

[34] Parse R. Hope: an international human becoming perspective. Sudbury (MA): Jones and Bartlett; 1999.

[35] Toomey A, Alligood M. Nursing theorists and their work. 6th edition. St. Louis (MO): Mosby, Inc; 2002.

[36] Einstein A. quoted on page 3, New York: New York Post; 1972.

[37] Gribbin J. Schrodinger's kittens and the search for reality: solving the quantum mysteries. Boston: Little Brown & Co; 1995.

[38] Brekke M, Schultz E. Energy theories. In: Erickson H, editor. Modeling and role-modeling: a view from the client's world. Cedar Park (TX): Unicorns Unlimited Book Publishers; 2006. p. 37–8, 36, 44–52, 59–60, 39.

[39] Pert C. Molecules of emotion. The science behind mind-body medicine. New York (NY): Scribner; 1997. p. 276.

[40] Ader R. Psychoneuroimmunology. New York: Academic Press; 1981.

[41] Erickson H, editor. Modeling and role-modeling: a view from the client's world. Cedar Park (TX): Unicorns Unlimited Book Publishers; 2006:62(107). p. 78–91.

[42] Walker M, Erickson H. Mind-body-spirit relations. In: Erickson H, editor. Modeling and role-modeling: a view from the client's world. Cedar Park (TX): Unicorns Unlimited Book Publishers; 2006. p. 67–94, 81–2, 68–94.

[43] Rogers M. Science of unitary human beings. In: Malinski VM, editor. Explorations of Martha Rogers' science of unitary human beings. Norwalk (CT): Appleton-Century-Crofts; 1986. p. 3–8.

[44] Krieger D. The therapeutic touch: how to use your hands to help or heal. New York: Fireside; 1979.

[45] Mentgen J. Healing touch. Nurs Clin North Am 2001;36(1):143–57.

[46] Mentgen J, Bulbrook MJ. Healing touch level I notebook. (NC): North Carolina Center for Healing Touch; 1994.

[47] For a more complete listing of modalities used by holistic nurses, visit the American Holistic Nurses Association Web site Available at: ahna@org.

[48] McKivergin M, Daubenmire M. The healing process of presence. J Holist Nurs 1994;12(1): 65–81.

[49] Dossey L. Healing words: the power of prayer and the practice of medicine. San Francisco (CA): HarperSanFrancisco; 1993.

[50] Kinney C. Heart-to-heart nurse-client relationships. In: Erickson H, editor. Modeling and role-modeling: a view from the client's world. (TX): Unicorns Unlimited Book Publishers; 2006. p. 284, 424–5.

[51] Kaliscchuk R, Davies B. A theory of healing in the aftermath of youth suicide. J Holist Nurs. 2001;19(2):163.

[52] McTaggart L. The field: the quest for the secret force of the universe. New York (NY): HarperCollins; 2002. p. 181, 194.

[53] Erickson H. Connecting. In: Erickson H, editor. Modeling and role-modeling: a view from the client's world. Cedar Park (TX): Unicorns Unlimited Book Publishers; 2006. p. 304, 309–17.

[54] Erickson H. The healing process. In: Erickson H, editor. Modeling and role-modeling: a view from the client's world. Cedar Park (TX): Unicorns Unlimited Book Publishers; 2006. p. 414.

[55] Erickson M. Developmental processes. In: Erickson H, editor. Modeling and role-modeling: a view from the client's world. Cedar Park (TX): Unicorns Unlimited Book Publishers; 2006. p. 179.

[56] McKivergin M. The nurse as an instrument of healing. In: Holistic nursing: a handbook for practice. 3rd edition. Gaithersburg (MD): Aspen Publishers, Inc.; 2000. p. 205–25.

[57] Rew L. Self reflections: consulting the truth within. In: Holistic nursing: a handbook for practice. 3rd edition. Gaithersburg (MD): Aspen Publishers, Inc.; 2000. p. 405–22.

[58] Erickson H. Facilitating development. In: Erickson H, editor. Modeling and role-modeling: a view from the client's world. Cedar Park (TX): Unicorns Unlimited Book Publishers; 2006. p. 354–5, 424.

[59] Watson J. Watson's theory of transpersonal caring. In: Walker PJ, Neuman B, editors. Blueprint for use of nursing models: education, research, practice and administration. New York: National League for Nursing Press; 1996. p. 141–84.

[60] Parse R. Scholarly dialogue: theory guides research and practice. Nurs Sci Q 1993;6:12.

[61] Patterson J, Zderad L. Humanistic nursing. (NLN Publ. No. 41–2218). New York: NLN Press; 1988.

[62] Watson J. Nursing science and nursing care. Norwalk (CT): Appleton-Century-Crofts; 1999.

[63] Parse R. Human becoming: Parse's theory of nursing. Nurs Sci Q 1992;5:35–42.

[64] Covington H. Caring presence: delineation of a concept for holistic nursing. J Holist Nurs. 2003;304–6.

[65] Chopra D. The seven spiritual laws of success. San Rafael (CA): New World Library and Amber-Allen Publishing; 1994.

[66] Waters P, Daubenmire M. Therapeutic capacity: the critical variance. In: Kritek P, editor. Reflections on healing: a central nursing construct. New York (NY): NLN Press; 1997. p. 56–68.

[67] Erickson H. Nurturing growth. In: Erickson H, editor. Modeling and role-modeling: a view from the client's world. Cedar Park (TX): Unicorns Unlimited Book Publishers; 2006. p. 342.

[68] Gerber R. Vibrational medicine for the 21st century. New York: HarperCollins; 2000. p. 470.

[69] Moss R. The I that is we. Millbrae (CA): Celestial Arts; 1981.

[70] Newman M. Health as expanding consciousness. St. Louis (MO): The C.V. Mosby Co.; 1986. p. 102–3, 3–4.

[71] Childre D, Martin H. The heartmath solution. San Francisco (CA): Harper-Collins Publishers; 1999.

[72] Keegan L, Dossey B. Profiles of nurse healers. New York (NY): Delmar Publishers; 1998. p. 5.

[73] Steere D. Spiritual presence in psychotherapy. New York (NY): Brunner/Mazel; 1997. p. 83.

[74] Erickson H. Searching for life purpose: discovering meaning. In: Erickson H, editor. Modeling and role-modeling: a view from the client's world. Cedar Park (TX): Unicorns Unlimited Book Publishers; 2006. p. 5–8, 5–32, 6–10.

[75] Parse R. Community: a human becoming perspective. Sudbury (MA): Jones & Bartlett; 2003.

[76] Emblen J, Pesut B. Strengthening transcendent meaning. J Holist Nurs 2001;19(1):42–56.

[77] Clayton D, Erickson H, Rogers S. Finding meaning in our life journey. In: Erickson H, editor. Modeling and role-modeling: a view from the client's world. Cedar Park (TX): Unicorns Unlimited Book Publishers; 2006. p. 392.

[78] Rew L. Self-reflection: consulting the truth within 2000. In: Dossey B, Keegan L, Guzetta C, editors. Holistic nursing: a handbook for practice. 4th edition. Boston: Jones and Bartlett Publishers; 2005. p. 407–23.

ELSEVIER
SAUNDERS

Nurs Clin N Am 42 (2007) 165–188

NURSING
CLINICS
OF NORTH AMERICA

Holistic Nursing as a Specialty: Holistic Nursing—Scope and Standards of Practice

Carla Mariano, EdD, RN, AHN-BC, FAAIM[a,b,*]

[a]Advanced Adult Holistic Nurse Practitioner Program, New York University, College of Nursing, 246 Greene Street, New York, NY 10003, USA
[b]American Holistic Nurses Association, AHNA National Office, 323 N. San Francisco Street, Suite 201, Flagstaff, AZ 86001, USA

Extraordinary changes have occurred in health care and nursing during the past decade. During this time holistic nurses recognized that not only were they practicing a unique specialty within nursing but also they needed to develop and publish a scope and standards of practice to document and define that specialty practice. The current *Holistic Nursing: Scope and Standards* (AHNA, 2007) documenting holistic practice was written to inform holistic nurses, the nursing profession, other health care providers and disciplines, employers, third-party payers, legislators, and the public about the unique scope of knowledge and the standards of practice and professional performance of a holistic nurse. The current standards are an updating and substantive revision of previous standards disseminated through the American Holistic Nurses Association (AHNA) [1,2]. Holistic Nursing was officially recognized as a specialty by the American Nurses Association (ANA) in November, 2006.

According to the ANA specialty standards are

...authoritative statements by which the nursing profession describes the responsibilities for which its practitioners are accountable. Consequently, standards reflect the values and priorities of the profession. Standards provide direction for professional nursing practice and a framework for evaluation of this practice. Written in measurable terms, these standards

---

Portions of the text are published in American Nurses Association, American Holistic Nurses Association. Holistic nursing: Scope and standards of practice. Washington, DC; 2007; reprinted with permission. Available at: www.ahna.org.

* 4 Washington Square Village, Apartment 5T, New York, NY 10012.
E-mail address: cm2@nyu.edu

define the nursing profession's accountability to the public and the outcomes for which registered nurses are responsible [3].

The current *Holistic Nursing: Scope and Standards of Practice* present a differentiation between practice at the basic and advanced-practice levels. The *Scope and Standards* are organized according to the criteria the ANA uses in recognizing a nursing specialty area [4,5] and build on nursing knowledge, skills, and competencies required for licensure. They provide a blueprint for holistic practice, education, and research.

Because holistic nursing emphasizes that human experiences are subjectively described and that health/illness is determined by the view of the individual, the *Scope and Standards* are derived from values that are central to the specialty and are consistent with the philosophies and theories of holism.

The purposes of this article are to discuss holistic nursing as a specialty, emphasizing its focus, knowledge base, and the context of its practices, to define holistic nursing's core values, to present information on the *Scope and Standards* of practice that guide nurses in this specialty, and to discuss the educational preparation of holistic nurses and the requirements for continued competence and currency in the field.

Scope of holistic nursing [6]

Holistic nursing as a nursing specialty

Holistic nursing is defined as "all nursing practice that has healing the whole person as its goal" [7]. Holistic nursing is a specialty practice that draws on nursing knowledge, theories of nursing, and wholeness, expertise, and intuition to guide nurses in becoming therapeutic partners with people in strengthening human responses to facilitate the healing process and achieve wholeness. Holistic nursing focuses on protecting, promoting, and optimizing health and wellness, assisting healing, preventing illness and injury, alleviating suffering, and supporting people to find peace, comfort, harmony, and balance through the diagnosis and treatment of human response.

In some sense, all nursing practice can be comprehensive—that is, all nursing practice may have a biopsychosocial perspective. What makes holistic nursing practice a specialty is that there is a philosophy, a body of knowledge, and an advanced set of nursing skills applied to practice that recognize the totality of the human being, the interconnectedness of body, mind, emotion, spirit, energy, social/cultural, relationship, context, and environment. Philosophically, holistic nursing is a world view, a way of being in the world, not just a modality. This philosophy honors the unique humanness of all people regardless of who and what they are. Knowledge for holistic nursing practice derives not only from nursing but also from theories of wholeness, energy, and unity, and from other healing systems and approaches. Holistic nurses incorporate conventional nursing and complementary/alternative modalities (CAM) and interventions into practice.

Through unconditional presence and intention, holistic nurses create environments conducive to healing, using techniques that promote empowerment, peace, comfort, and a subjective sense of harmony and well-being for the person. The holistic nurse acts in partnership with the individual or family in providing options and alternatives regarding health and treatment. Additionally, the holistic nurse assists the person to find meaning in the health/illness experience.

Holistic nursing focuses on integrating simultaneously as an iterative process all of these realms (ie, a philosophy of being and living, using theories of nursing and wholeness with related knowledge and skills, focusing on the unity and totality of humans, incorporating healing approaches, creating healing environments, partnering and empowering individuals and assisting in the exploration of meaning in the care of people). In holistic nursing, the nurse is the facilitator of healing, honoring that the person heals him- or herself. The holistic nurse assists individuals to identify themselves as the healer and access their own innate healing capacities.

The practice of holistic nursing requires nurses to integrate self-care and self-responsibility into their own lives, serving as a role model for others. They strive for an awareness of the interconnectedness of individuals to the human and global community. Holistic nurses thus also attend to the health of the ecosystem.

The holistic nurse is an instrument of healing and a facilitator in the healing process. Holistic nurses honor the individual's subjective experience about health, health beliefs, and values. To become therapeutic partners with individuals, families, communities, and populations, holistic nursing practice draws on nursing knowledge, theories, research, expertise, intuition, and creativity incorporating the roles of clinician, educator, consultant, partner, role model, and advocate. Holistic nursing practice encourages peer review of professional practice in various clinical settings and provides care based on current professional standards, laws, and regulations governing nursing practice. The major phenomena of concern to holistic nursing are listed in Box 1.

The core values of holistic nursing: integrating the art and science

Holistic nursing emanates from five core values summarizing the ideals and principles of the specialty. These core values are:

1. Philosophy, Theory, and Ethics
2. Holistic Caring Process
3. Holistic Communication, Therapeutic Environment, and Cultural Diversity
4. Holistic Education and Research
5. Holistic Nurse Self-Care

Each of these core values is discussed below.

Box 1. Phenomena of concern to holistic nursing

The caring–healing relationship
The subjective experience of and meanings ascribed to health,
    illness, wellness, healing, birth, growth and development, and
    dying
The cultural values and beliefs and folk practices of health,
    illness, and healing
Spirituality in nursing care
The evaluation of alternative/complementary modalities used in
    nursing practice
Comprehensive health promotion and disease prevention
Self-care processes
Physical, mental, emotional, and spiritual comfort, discomfort,
    and pain
Empowerment, decision-making, and the ability to make
    informed choices
Social and economic policies and their effects on the health of
    individuals, families, and communities
Diverse and alternative health care systems and their
    relationships with access and quality of health care
The environment and the prevention of disease

From American Nurses Association, American Holistic Nurses Association.
Holistic nursing: Scope and standards of practice. Washington, DC; 2007.

Holistic philosophy, theory, and ethics

Holistic nurses recognize the human health experience as a complicated, dynamic relationship of health, illness, and wellness and value healing as the desired outcome of the practice of nursing. Their practice is based on scientific foundations (theory, research, evidence-based practice, critical thinking, reflection) and art (relationship, communication, creativity, presence, caring). Holistic nursing is grounded in nursing knowledge and skill and guided by nursing theory. Although each holistic nurse chooses which nursing theory to apply in any individual case, the nursing theories of Florence Nightingale, Jean Watson (the *Theory of Human Caring*), Martha Rogers (the *Science of Unitary Human Beings*), Margaret Newman (*Health as Expanding Consciousness*), Madeline Leininger (*Theory of Cultural Care*), Rosemarie Rizzo Parse (*Theory of Human Becoming*), Paterson and Zderad (*Humanistic Nursing Theory*), and Helen Erickson (*Modeling and Role-Modeling*) are most frequently used to support holistic nursing practice.

In addition to nursing theory, holistic nurses use other theories and perspectives of wholeness and healing to guide their practice. These scientific theories and philosophies present a world view of connectedness (eg, Theories of Consciousness; Energy Field Theory; C. Pribram's Holographic Universe; D. Bohm's Implicate/Explicate Order; C. Pert's Psychoneuroimmunology; K. Wilbur's Spectrum of Consciousness and Integral Psychology; Spirituality; and Alternative Medical Systems, such as Traditional Oriental Medicine, Ayurveda, Native American and Indigenous Healing, and Eastern Contemplative orientations, such as Zen and Taoism).

Holistic nurses further recognize and honor the ethic that the person is the authority on his or her own health experience. The holistic nurse is an "option giver," helping the person develop an understanding of alternatives and implications of various health and treatment options. The holistic nurse first ascertains what the individual thinks or believes is happening to him or her and then assists the person to identify what will help his or her situation. The assessment begins from where the individual is. The holistic nurse then discusses options, including the person's choices, across a continuum, and possible effects and implications of each. For instance, if a person diagnosed with cancer is experiencing nausea due to chemotherapy, the individual and nurse may discuss the choices and effects of pharmacologic agents, imagery, homeopathic remedies, and so forth, or a combination of these. The holistic nurse acts as partner and co-prescriptor versus sole prescriber. The relationship is a copiloting of the individual's health experience whereby the nurse respects the person's decision about his or her own health. It is a process of engagement versus compliance.

Client narratives, whether they arise from individuals, families, or communities, provide the context of the experiences and are used as an important focus in understanding the person's situation. Holistic nurses hold the belief that people, through their inherent capacities, heal themselves. The holistic nurse therefore is not the healer but the guide and facilitator of the individual's own healing.

In the belief that all things are connected, the holistic perspective espouses that an individual's actions have a ripple effect throughout humanity. Holism places the greatest worth on individuals' developing higher levels of human awareness. This, in turn, elevates the whole of humanity. Holistic nurses believe in the sacredness of one's self and of all nature. One's inner self and the collective greater self have stewardship not only over one's body, mind, and spirit, but also over our planet. Holistic nurses focus on the meaning and quality of life deriving from their own character and from their relationship to the universe rather than imposed from without.

Holistic nurses hold to a professional ethic of caring and healing that seeks to preserve wholeness and dignity of self and others. They support human dignity by advocating and adhering to the *Patient's Bill of Rights* [8], the *ANA Code of Ethics with Interpretive Standards* [9] and *The AHNA Position Statement on Holistic Nursing Ethics* [10].

Holistic caring process

Holistic nurses provide care that recognizes the totality of the human being (the interconnectedness of body, mind, emotion, spirit, social/cultural, relationship, context, and environment). This is an integrated and comprehensive approach. While physical symptoms are being treated, a holistic nurse would also focus on how the individual is cognitively perceiving and emotionally dealing with the illness, its effect on the person's family and social relationships and economic resources, the person's values and cultural or spiritual beliefs and preferences regarding treatment, and the meaning of this experience to the person's life. But in addition, holistic nurses may also incorporate a number of modalities (eg, cognitive restructuring, stress management, visualization, aroma therapy, therapeutic touch) with conventional nursing interventions. Holistic nurses focus on care interventions that promote healing, peace, comfort, and a subjective sense of well-being for the person.

The holistic caring process involves six often simultaneously occurring steps: assessment, diagnosis (pattern/problem/need identification), outcomes, therapeutic plan of care, implementation, and evaluation. Holistic nurses apply the holistic caring process with individuals, families across the life span, population groups, and communities, and in all settings.

Holistic nurses incorporate a variety of roles in their practice, including expert clinician and facilitator of healing; consultant and collaborator; educator and guide; administrator, leader, and change agent; researcher; and advocate. They strongly emphasize partnership with individuals throughout the entire decision-making process.

Holistic assessments include not only the physical, functional, psychosocial, mental, emotional, cultural, and sexual aspects but also the spiritual, transpersonal, and energy-field assessments of the whole person. Energy assessments are based on the concept that all beings are composed of energy. Congestion or stagnation of energy in any realm creates dis-harmony and dis-ease. Spiritual assessments glean not only religious beliefs and practices but query about a person's meaning and purpose in life and how that may have changed because of the present health experience. Spiritual assessments also include questions about an individual's sense of serenity and peace, what provides joy and fulfillment, and the source of strength and hope. Holistic assessment data are interpreted into patterns/challenges/needs from which meaning and understanding of the health/disease experience can be mutually identified with the person. An important responsibility is that of helping the person to identify risk factors, such as lifestyle, habits, beliefs and values, personal and family health history, and age-related conditions, that influence health and then to use opportunities to increase well-being. The focus is on the individual's goals, not those of the nurse.

Therapeutic plans of care respect the person's experience and the uniqueness of each healing journey. The same illness may have very different manifestations in different individuals. A major aspect of holistic nursing practice, in addition to competence, is intention. That is, intending for the wholeness, well-being, and highest good of the person with every encounter and intervention. This honors and reinforces the innate capacity of people to heal themselves. Holistic nurses therefore respect that outcomes may not be what is expected and may evolve differently based on the person's own individual healing process and health choices. Holistic nurses endeavor to detach themselves from the outcomes. The nurse does not produce the outcomes; the individual's own healing process produces the outcomes and the nurse facilitates this process. A significant focus is on guiding individuals and significant others to use their own inner strength and resources through the course of healing.

Appropriate and evidence-based information (including current knowledge, practice, and research) regarding the health condition and various treatments and therapies and their side effects is consistently provided. Holistic care always occurs within the scope and standards of practice of registered nursing and in accordance with state and federal laws and regulations.

Therapies frequently incorporated in holistic nursing practice include the following interventions: meditation; relaxation therapy; breath work; music, art, and aroma therapies; energy-based touch therapies, such as therapeutic touch, healing touch, Reiki; acupressure; massage; guided imagery; animal-assisted therapy; biofeedback; prayer; reflexology; hypnosis; diet; herbology; and homeopathy. Interventions frequently employed in holistic nursing practice in addition to conventional nursing interventions include anxiety reduction and stress management, calming technique, emotional support, exercise and nutrition promotion, smoking cessation, patient contracting, resiliency promotion, forgiveness facilitation, hope installation, presence, journaling, counseling, cognitive therapy, self-help, spiritual support, and environmental management [11].

Because many of today's health care problems are stress related, holistic nurses empower individuals by teaching them techniques to reduce their stress. Many interventions used in holistic nursing elicit the relaxation response (eg, breath work, meditation, relaxation, imagery, aromatherapy and essential oils, diet). People can learn these therapies and use them without the intervention of a health care provider. This allows people to take an active role in the management of their own health care. Holistic nurses also can teach families and caregivers to use these techniques for loved ones who may be ill (eg, simple foot or hand massage for older clients with dementia). In addition, individuals are taught how to evaluate their own responses to these modalities.

Holistic nurses prescribe as legally authorized. They instruct individuals regarding drug, herbal, and homeopathic regimens and importantly the side effects and interactions between, for example, medications and herbs. They consult, collaborate, and refer as necessary, to both conventional allopathic providers and to holistic practitioners. They provide information and counseling to people about alternative, complementary, integrative, and conventional health care practices. Very importantly holistic nurses facilitate negotiation of services as they guide individuals and families between conventional western medical and alternative systems. Holistic nurses, in partnership with the individual and others, evaluate if care is effective and if there are changes in the meaning of the health experience for the individual.

Holistic communication, therapeutic environment, and cultural diversity

The holistic nurse's communication ensures that each individual experiences the presence of the nurse as authentic, caring, compassionate, and sincere. This is more than therapeutic techniques, such as responding, reflecting, summarizing, and so forth. This is deep listening, or as some say, "listening with the heart and not just the ears." It is done with conscious intention and without preconceptions, busyness, distractions, or analysis. It takes place in the "now" within an atmosphere of shared humanness, human being to human being. Through presence or "being within the moment," holistic nurses provide each person with an interpersonal encounter that is experienced as a connection with one who is giving undivided attention to the needs and concerns of the individual. Using unconditional positive regard, holistic nurses convey to the individual receiving care the belief in his or her worth and value as a human being, not solely the recipient of medical and nursing interventions.

The importance of context in understanding the person's health experience is always recognized. Space and time are allowed for exploration. Each person's health encounter is truly seen as unique and may be contrary to conventional knowledge and treatments. The holistic nurse must therefore be comfortable with ambiguity, paradox, and uncertainty. This requires a perspective that the nurse is not "the expert" regarding another's health/illness experience.

Holistic nurses have a knowledge base of the use and meanings of symbolic language and use interventions, such as imagery, creation of sacred space and personal rituals, dream exploration, and aesthetic therapies, such as music, visual arts, and dance. They encourage and support others in the use of prayer, meditation, or other spiritual and symbolic practices for healing purposes.

A cornerstone of holistic nursing practice is assisting individuals to find meaning in their experience. Regardless of the health/illness condition, the meaning that individuals ascribe to their situation can influence their response to it. Holistic nurses attend to the subjective world of the individual. They consider meanings, such as the person's concerns in relation to health, family economics, as well as to deeper meanings related to the person's purpose in life. Regardless of the technology or treatment, holistic nurses address the human spirit as a major force in healing. The person's perception of meaning is related to all factors in health–wellness–disease–illness.

Holistic nurses realize that suffering, illness, and disease are natural components of the human condition and have the potential to teach us about ourselves, our relationships, and our universe. Every experience is valued for its meaning and lesson.

Holistic nurses have a particular obligation to create a therapeutic environment that values holism, caring, social support, and integration of conventional and CAM approaches to healing. They seek to create environments where individuals, both clients and staff, feel connected, supported, and respected. A particular perspective of holistic nursing is the nurse as the "healing environment" and an instrument of healing. Holistic nurses shape the physical environment (eg, light, fresh air, pleasant sounds or quiet, neatness and order, healing smells, earth elements). They also provide a relationship-focused environment (ie, creation of sacred space through presence and intention where another can feel safe, can unfold, can explore the dimensions of self in healing).

Culture, beliefs, and values are inherent components of a holistic approach. Concepts of health and healing are based in culture and often influence people's actions to promote, maintain, and restore health. Culture also may provide an understanding of a person's concept of the illness or disease and appropriate treatment. Holistic nurses possess knowledge and understanding of numerous cultural traditions and health care practices from various racial, ethnic, and social backgrounds. Holistic nurses honor the individual's understanding and articulation of his or her own cultural values, beliefs, and health practices versus reliance on stereotypical cultural classifications and descriptions. These understandings then are used to provide culturally competent care that corresponds with the beliefs, values, traditions, and health practices of people. Holistic nurses ask individuals "what do I need to know about you culturally in caring for you?"

Holistic healing is a collaborative approach. Holistic nurses take an active role in trying to remove the political and financial barriers to the inclusion of holistic care in the health care system.

Of particular importance to holistic nurses is the human connection with the ecology. They actively participate in building an ecosystem that sustains the well-being of all life. This includes raising the public's consciousness about environmental issues and stressors that affect not only the health of people but the health of the planet.

Holistic education and research

Holistic nurses have a richness as part of their formal academic and continuing education. They possess an understanding of a wide range of cultural norms, health care practices/beliefs/values concerning individuals, families, groups, and communities from varied racial, ethnic, spiritual, and social background. This knowledge base also includes a wide diversity of practices and modalities outside of conventional medicine. Because of this holistic nurses have a significant impact on peoples' understanding of health care options and alternatives, thus serving as both educators and advocates.

Additionally, holistic nurses provide much-needed information to individuals on health promotion, including such topics as healthy lifestyles, risk-reducing behaviors, preventive self-care, stress management, living with changes secondary to illness and treatment, and opportunities to enhance well-being.

Holistic nurses value all the ways of knowing and learning. They individualize learning and appreciate that science, intuition, introspection, creativity, aesthetics, and culture produce different bodies of knowledge and perspectives. They help others to know themselves and access their inner wisdom to enhance growth, wholeness, and well-being.

Holistic nurses often guide individuals and families in their health care decisions, especially regarding conventional allopathic and complementary/alternative practices. They must be knowledgeable about the best evidence available for both conventional and CAM therapies. In addition to developing evidence-based practice using research, practice guidelines, and expertise, holistic nurses strongly consider the person's values and health care practices and beliefs in practice decisions.

Holistic nurses look at alternative philosophies of science and research methods that are compatible with investigations of humanistic and holistic occurrences; that explore the context in which phenomena occur and the meaning of patterns that evolve; and that take into consideration the interactive nature of the body, mind, emotion, spirit, and environment.

Holistic nurses conduct and evaluate research in diverse areas such as:

Outcome measures of various holistic therapies (eg, therapeutic touch, prayer, aroma therapy)

Instrument development to measure caring behaviors and dimensions; spirituality; self-transcendence; cultural competence, and so forth

Client responses to holistic interventions in health/illness

Explorations of clients lived experiences with various health/illness phenomena

Theory development in healing, caring, intentionality, cultural constructions, empowerment and so forth

Further, research that advances the work of holistic nursing theories (Watson, Erickson, Rogers, Newman, Parse, and Leininger) helps to build the knowledge base of nursing and advance the nursing science of holism. AHNA has incorporated an active research agenda by assisting and mentoring members in research endeavors, granting research awards, identifying and reporting on research that focuses on holistic healing phenomena and modalities, and applying research in practice.

Holistic nurse self-care

Self-care, personal awareness of, and continuous focus on being an instrument of healing are significant requirements for holistic nurses. Holistic nurses value themselves and mobilize the necessary resources to care for themselves. They endeavor to integrate self-awareness, self-care, and self-healing into their lives by incorporating practices such as self-assessment, meditation, yoga, good nutrition, energy therapies, movement, art, support, and lifelong learning. Holistic nurses honor their unique patterns and the development of the body, the psychological–social–cultural self, the intellectual self, and the spiritual self. Nurses cannot facilitate healing unless they are in the process of healing themselves. Through continuing education, practice, and self-work, holistic nurses develop the skills of authentic and deep self-reflection and introspection to understand themselves and their journey. It is seen as a lifelong process.

Holistic nurses strive to achieve harmony/balance in their own lives and assist others to do the same. They create healing environments for themselves by attending to their own well-being, letting go of self-destructive behaviors and attitudes, practicing centering and stress-reduction techniques. By doing this, holistic nurses serve as role models to others, be they clients, colleagues, or personal relations.

Standards of holistic nursing practice [6]

Overarching philosophical principles of holistic nursing

Holistic nurses express, contribute to, and promote an understanding of a philosophy of nursing that values healing as the desired outcome; the human health experience as a complex, dynamic relationship of health, illness, disease and wellness; the scientific foundations of nursing practice; and nursing as an art. It is based on the following overarching philosophical tenets which are embedded in every standard of practice.

Principles of holistic nursing

The following principles underlie holistic nursing:

Person

There is unity, totality, and connectedness of everyone and everything
(body, mind, emotion, spirit, sexuality, age, environment, social/
cultural, belief systems, relationships, context).
Human beings are unique and inherently good.
People are able to find meaning and purpose in their own life, experiences, and illness.
All people have an innate power and capacity for self-healing. Health/
illness is subjectively described and determined by the view of the

individual. The person therefore is honored in all phases of his/her healing process regardless of expectations or outcomes.

People/person/individuals identify (are) the recipient of holistic nursing services. These can be clients, patients, families, significant others, populations or communities. They may be ill and within the health care delivery system or well, moving toward personal betterment to enhance well-being.

Healing/health

Health and illness are natural and a part of life, learning, and movement toward change and development.

Health is seen as balance, integration, harmony, right relationship, and the betterment of well-being, not just the absence of disease. Healing can take place without cure. The focus is on health promotion/disease prevention/ health restoration/lifestyle patterns and habits and symptom relief.

Illness is considered a teacher and an opportunity for self-awareness and growth as part of the life process. Symptoms are respected as messages.

People, as active partners in the healing process, are empowered when they take some control of their own lives, health, and well-being, including personal choices and relationships.

Treatment is a process that considers the root of the problem, not merely treating the obvious signs and symptoms.

Practice

Practice is a science (critical thinking, evidence/research/theory as underlying practice) and an art (intuition, creativity, presence, self/personal knowing as integral to practice).

The values and ethic of holism, caring, moral insight, dignity, integrity, competence, responsibility, accountability, and legality underline holistic nursing practice.

There are various philosophies and paradigms of health, illness, healing, and approaches/models for the delivery of health care in the United States and in other cultures that need to be understood and used.

Older adults represent the predominant population served by nurses.

Public policy and the health care delivery system influence the health and well-being of society and professional nursing.

Nursing roles

The nurse is part of the healing environment using warmth, compassion, caring, authenticity, respect, trust, and relationship as instruments of healing in and of themselves.

Using conventional nursing interventions and holistic/complementary/ alternative/integrative modalities that enhance the body–mind–emotion–spirit connectedness to foster healing, health, wholeness, and well-being of people.

Collaborating, and partnering with all constituencies in the health process including the person receiving care and family, community, peers, and other disciplines. Using principles and skills of cooperation, alliance, and respect, and honoring the contributions of all.

Participating in the change process to develop more caring cultures in which to practice and learn.

Assisting nurses to nurture and heal themselves.

Participating in activities that contribute to the improvement of communities, the environment, and the betterment of public health.

Acting as an advocate for the rights of and equitable distribution and access to health care for all people, especially vulnerable populations.

Honoring the ecosystem and our relationship with and need to preserve it because we are all connected.

Self-care

The nurse's self-reflection and self-assessment, self-care, healing, and personal development are necessary for service to others and growth/change in one's own well-being and understanding of one's own personal journey.

The nurse values oneself and one's calling to holistic nursing as a life purpose.

Holistic nursing practice is guided by the holistic caring process, whether used with individuals, families, population groups, or communities. This process involves assessment, diagnosis, outcome identification, planning, implementation and evaluation. It encompasses all significant actions taken in providing culturally, ethically, respectful, compassionate, and relevant holistic nursing care to all persons.

The standards of holistic nursing practice

There are 15 Standards for ANA recognition as a nursing specialty, 6 for practice and 9 for professional performance; thus there are 15 standards for holistic nursing. Each standard addresses measurement criteria for both the registered nurse and the advanced practice nurse. These standards and examples of measurement criteria (as each standard has numerous measurement criteria) are found in Appendix 1.

Educational preparation and certification for holistic nursing practice [6]

Holistic nurses are registered nurses who are educationally prepared for practice from an approved school of nursing and are licensed to practice in their individual state, commonwealth, or territory. The holistic registered nurse's experience, education, knowledge, and abilities establish the level of competence. *Holistic Nursing: Scope and Standards of Practice,* (2007) identifies the scope of practice of holistic nursing and the specific standards and associated measurement criteria of holistic nurses at both the basic and advanced levels. Regardless of the level of practice, all holistic nurses integrate the previously identified five core values.

A registered nurse may prepare for the specialty of holistic nursing in a variety of ways. Educational offerings range from baccalaureate and graduate courses and programs, to continuing education programs with extensive contact hours.

Basic practice level

The education of all nursing students preparing for RN licensure includes basic content on physiological, psychological, emotional, and some spiritual processes with populations across the lifespan and conventional nursing care practices within each of these domains. Additionally, basic nursing education incorporates experiences in a variety of clinical/practice settings from acute care to community. The educational focus is most frequently on "specialties," however, often emanating from the biomedical disease model/cure orientation. In holistic nursing, the individual across the lifespan is viewed in context as an integrated body, mind, emotion, social, spirit totality, with the emphasis on wholeness, well-being, health promotion, and healing using both conventional and complementary/alternative practices. Because of the lack of intentional focus on integration, unity, and healing, the educational exposure of most nursing students is not adequate preparation for assuming the specialty role of a holistic nurse.

A number of schools of nursing are beginning to incorporate holistic nursing content at the undergraduate level, whether it be as discrete courses, such as therapeutic touch, relaxation, aromatherapy, and so forth, or integrated in courses such as nursing therapeutics.

Advanced practice level

As with the basic level, there are a variety of ways (both academic and professional development) in which registered nurses can acquire the additional specialized knowledge and skills that prepare them for practice as an advanced practice holistic nurse. These nurses are expected to hold a master's or doctoral degree and demonstrate a greater depth and scope of knowledge, a greater integration of information, increased complexity of skills and interventions, and notable role autonomy. They provide leadership in practice, teaching, research, consultation, advocacy, and/or policy formation in advancing holistic nursing to improve the holistic health of people [6]. Several schools of nursing that offer graduate programs in holistic nursing have a stable or growing number of applicants. In addition, there are numerous continuing education offerings in holistic nursing care and several certificate programs throughout the country focus on specific modalities and on the essence of holism.

Continuing education for both basic and advanced practice levels

The American Holistic Nurses Association (AHNA) is a provider and approver of continuing education, recognized by the American Nurses Credentialing Center (ANCC). Continuing educational programs, workshops and lectures in holistic nursing and CAM have been popular nationwide, with AHNA or other bodies granting continuing education units.

AHNA endorses certificate programs in specific areas. These include Spirituality, Health and Healing, Reflexology; Imagery, Aromatherapy, Healing Touch, Amma Therapy, Clinical Nursing Assessment, and Whole Health Education. It also approves continuing education offerings in holistic nursing as well as giving the AHNA home study course, Foundation of Holistic Nursing. Other programs in distinct therapies, like acupuncture, Reiki, homeopathy, massage, imagery, healing arts, holistic health, Oriental Medicine, nutrition, Ayurveda, therapeutic touch, healing touch, herbology, chiropractic, and so forth, are given nationally as degrees, certificates, or continuing education programs by centers, specialty organizations or schools [6].

Certification

Competency mechanisms for evaluating holistic nursing practice as a specialty exist through a national certification/recertification process overseen by the American Holistic Nurses Certification Corporation (AHNCC). The AHNCC certifies at the basic level (HN-BC) which requires a baccalaureate degree and the advanced practice level (AHN-BC) which requires a graduate degree in nursing. Further, the AHNCC provides endorsement for schools of nursing meeting the standards of holistic nursing practice. Additionally, holistic nurses often are certified in specific CAM modalities, such as Imagery, Reiki, Aromatherapy, Healing Touch, Biofeedback, and Reflexology.

Settings for holistic nursing practice [6]

Holistic nurses practice in numerous settings, including but not limited to: private practitioner offices; ambulatory, acute, long-term, and home care settings; complementary care centers; women's health centers; hospice palliative care; psychiatric mental health facilities; schools; rehabilitation centers; community nursing organizations; student and employee health; managed care organizations; independent self-employed practice; correctional facilities; professional nursing and health care organizations; administration; staff development; and universities and colleges. Holistic nursing practice also occurs when there is a request for consultation or when holistic nurses advocate for care that promotes health, prevents disease, illness, or disability for individuals, communities, or the environment (ie, a holistic nurse may choose not to work in a critical care setting but provide consultation regarding self-care or stress management to nurses in that area). Or, holistic nurses may practice in preoperative and recovery rooms instituting a "Prepare for

Surgery" program that teaches individuals having surgery meditation and positive affirmation techniques, pre and post surgery while incorporating a homeopathic regimen for trauma and cell healing. Employment or voluntary participation of holistic nurses also can influence civic activities and the regulatory and legislative arena at the local, state, national, or international level.

As holistic nursing focuses on wellness, wholeness, and development of the whole person, holistic nurses also practice in health enhancement settings, such as spas, gyms, and wellness centers.

Because holistic nursing is a world view, way of "being" in the world, and not just a modality, holistic nurses can practice in any setting and with individuals throughout the life span. As the public increasingly requests holistic/CAM services, holistic nurses will be increasingly in demand and practice in a wider array of settings. Holistic nursing takes place wherever healing occurs.

Summary

The specialty practice of holistic nursing is generally not well understood. Each holistic nurse must therefore educate other nurses, health care providers and disciplines, and the public about the role, value, and benefits of holistic nursing, whether it be in direct practice, education, management, or research. Holistic nurses articulate the ideas underpinning the holistic paradigm and the philosophy of the caring–healing model. Jean Watson reminds us that society and the public are searching for something deeper in terms of realizing self-care, self-knowledge, and self-healing potentials. Nurses need to acknowledge the human aspects of practice—attending to people and their experience rather that just focusing on the medical orientation and disease. She concludes that "nurses have a covenant with the public to sustain caring. It is our collective responsibility to transform caring practices into the framework that identifies and gives distinction to nursing as a profession" [12]. The publication and dissemination of the *Holistic Nursing: Scope and Standards of Practice* are a means through which holistic nurses are educating the profession about the values, principles and practice requirements of the specialty.

Appendix 1 [6]

Standard 1. ASSESSMENT: The holistic nurse collects comprehensive data pertinent to the person's health or situation.

The holistic registered nurse:

- Collects comprehensive data including but not limited to physical, functional, psychosocial, emotional, mental, sexual, cultural, age-related, environmental, spiritual/transpersonal and energy field assessments in a systematic and ongoing process while honoring the uniqueness of the person.

- Identifies areas such as the person's health and cultural practices, values, beliefs, preferences, meanings of health, illness, lifestyle patterns, family issues, and risk behaviors and context.

The holistic advanced practice registered nurse:

- Initiates and interprets diagnostic procedures relevant to the person's current status.
- Explores the meanings of the symbolic language expressing itself in areas such as dreams, images, symbols, sensations, prayers that are a part of the individual's health experience.

Standard 2. DIAGNOSIS OR HEALTH ISSUES: The holistic nurse analyzes the assessment data to determine the diagnosis or issues expressed as actual or potential patterns/problems/needs which are related to health, wellness, disease, or illness.

The holistic registered nurse:

- Derives the diagnosis or health issues based on holistic assessment data
- Assists the person to explore the meaning of the health/disease experience.

The holistic advanced practice registered nurse:

- Uses complex data and information obtained during interview, examination, and diagnostic procedures in identifying diagnosis.

Standard 3: OUTCOMES IDENTIFICATION: The holistic registered nurse identifies outcomes for a plan individualized to the person or the situation. The holistic nurse values the evolution and the process of healing as it unfolds. This implies that specific unfolding outcomes may not be evident immediately due to the non-linear nature of the healing process so that both expected/anticipated and evolving outcomes are considered.

The holistic registered nurse:

- Defines outcomes in terms of the person; the individual's values and beliefs, preferences, age, spiritual practices; ethical considerations, environment, or situation with such consideration as associated risks, benefits, and costs, and current scientific evidence.
- Partners with the person to identify realistic goals based on the person's present and potential capabilities and quality of life.

The holistic advanced practice registered nurse:

- Identifies outcomes that incorporate patient satisfaction, the person's understanding and meanings in their unique patterns and processes, quality of life, cost and clinical effectiveness, and continuity and consistency among providers.

Standard 4. PLANNING: The holistic registered nurse develops a plan that identifies strategies and alternatives to attain outcomes.

The holistic registered nurse:

- Develops in partnership with the person an individualized plan considering the person's characteristics or situation including but not limited to values, beliefs, spiritual and health practices, preferences, choices, age and cultural appropriateness, environmental sensitivity.
- Develops the plan in conjunction with the person, family, and others, as appropriate.
- Establishes practice settings and safe space and time for both the nurse and person, family/significant others to explore suggested, potential, and alternative options.

The holistic advanced practice registered nurse:

- Identifies assessment, diagnostic strategies, therapeutic interventions within the plan and including therapeutic effects and side effects that reflect current evidence, data, research, literature, and expert clinical knowledge and the person's experiences.
- Uses linguistic and symbolic language including but not limited to word associations, dreams, storytelling, journals to explore with individuals, possibilities, and options.

Standard 5. IMPLEMENTATION: The holistic registered nurse implements in partnership with the person the identified plan.

The holistic registered nurse:

- Partners with the person/family/significant others/caregiver to implement the plan in a safe and timely manner while honoring the person's choices and unique healing journey.

The holistic advanced practice registered nurse:

- Facilitates use of systems and community resources to implement the plan.
- Incorporates new knowledge and strategies to initiate change in nursing care practices if desired outcomes are not achieved.

Standard 5A: COORDINATION OF CARE: The holistic registered nurse coordinates care delivery.

The holistic registered nurse:

- Coordinates implementation of the plan.

The holistic advanced practice registered nurse:

- Provides leadership in the coordination of multidisciplinary health care for integrated delivery of person care services.

Standard 5B: HEALTH TEACHING AND HEALTH PROMOTION: The holistic registered nurse employs strategies to promote holistic health/wellness and a safe environment.

The holistic registered nurse:

- Provides health teaching to individuals, families, and significant others or caregivers that enhances the mind–body emotion–spirit connection.
- Uses health promotion and health teaching methods appropriate to the situation and the individual's values, beliefs, health practices, age, learning needs, readiness and ability to learn, language preference, spirituality, culture and socioeconomic status.
- Assists others to access their own inner wisdom, which may provide opportunities to enhance and support growth, development and wholeness.

The holistic advanced practice registered nurse:

- Synthesizes empirical evidence on risk behaviors, decision making about life choices, learning theories, behavioral change theories, motivational theories, epidemiology, and other related theories and frameworks when designing holistic health information and education.

Standard 5C: CONSULTATION: The holistic advanced practice registered nurse provides consultation to influence the identified plan, enhance the abilities of others, and effect change.

The holistic advanced practice registered nurse:

- Facilitates the effectiveness of a consultation by involving all stake holders including the individual in decision-making and negotiating role responsibilities.

Standard 5D: PRESCRIPTIVE AUTHORITY AND TREATMENT: The holistic advanced practice registered nurse uses prescriptive authority, procedures, referrals, treatments, and therapies in accordance with state and federal laws and regulations.

The holistic advanced practice registered nurse:

- Prescribes treatments, therapies, and procedures based on evidence, research, current knowledge, and practice considering the person's holistic health care needs and choices.
- Uses advanced knowledge of pharmacology, psychoneuroimmunology, nutritional supplements, herbal and homeopathic remedies, and a variety of complementary and alternative therapies in prescribing.
- Evaluates therapeutic and potential adverse effects of pharmacological and non-pharmacological treatments including but not limited to drug/

herbal/homeopathic regimens as well as drug/herbal/homeopathic side effects and interactions.

Standard 6: EVALUATION: The holistic registered nurse evaluates progress toward attainment of outcomes while recognizing and honoring the continuing holistic nature of the healing process.

The holistic registered nurse:

- Conducts a holistic, systematic, ongoing, and criterion-based evaluation of the outcomes in relation to the structures and processes prescribed by the plan and the indicated timeline.
- Evaluates in partnership with the person, the effectiveness of the planned strategies in relation to the person's responses and the attainment of the expected and unfolding outcomes.

The holistic advanced practice registered nurse:

- Uses the results of the evaluation analyses to make or recommend process or structural changes, including policy, procedure, and/or protocol documentation, as appropriate to improve holistic care.

Standard 7: QUALITY OF PRACTICE: The holistic registered nurse systematically enhances the quality and effectiveness of holistic nursing practice.

The holistic registered nurse:

- Participates in quality improvement activities for holistic nursing practice:

The holistic advanced practice registered nurse:

- Evaluates the practice environment and quality of holistic nursing care rendered in relation to existing evidence, feedback from individuals and significant others, identifying opportunities for the generation and use of research.

Standard 8: EDUCATION: The holistic registered nurse attains knowledge and competency that reflects current nursing practice.

The holistic registered nurse:

- Seeks experiences and formal and independent learning activities to maintain and develop clinical and professional skills and knowledge and personal growth to provide holistic care.

The holistic advanced practice registered nurse:

- Uses current health care research findings and other evidence to expand clinical knowledge, enhance role performance, and increase knowledge of professional issues and changes in national standards for practice and trends in holistic care.

Standard 9: PROFESSIONAL PRACTICE EVALUATION: The holistic registered nurse evaluates one's own nursing practice in relation to professional practice standards and guidelines, relevant statutes, rules, and regulations. The holistic registered nurse's practice reflects the application of knowledge of current practice standards, guidelines, statutes, rules, regulations.

The holistic registered nurse:

- Reflects on one's practice and how one's own personal, cultural, spiritual beliefs, experiences, biases, education and values may affect care given to individuals/families/communities.
- Engages in self-evaluation of practice on a regular basis, identifying areas of strength, as well as areas in which professional development and personal growth would be beneficial.

The holistic advanced practice registered nurse:

- Engages in a formal process, seeking feedback regarding one's own practice from individuals receiving care, peers, professional colleagues, and others.

Standard 10: COLLEGIALITY: The holistic registered nurse interacts with and contributes to the professional development of peers and colleagues.

The holistic registered nurse:

- Shares knowledge and skills with peers and colleagues as evidenced by such activities as patient care conferences or presentations at formal or informal meetings.
- Promotes work environments conductive to support, understanding, respect, health, healing, caring, wholeness, and harmony.

The holistic advanced practice registered nurse:

- Models expert holistic nursing practice to interdisciplinary team members and health care consumers.

Standard 11: COLLABORATION: The holistic registered nurse collaborates with the person, family, and others in the conduct of holistic nursing practice.

The holistic registered nurse:

- Communicates with the person, family, significant others, caregivers, and interdisciplinary health care providers regarding the person's care and the holistic nurse's role in the provision of that care.

The holistic advanced practice registered nurse:

- Facilitates the negotiation of holistic/complementary/integrative and conventional health care services for continuity of care and program planning.

Standard 12: ETHICS: The holistic registered nurse integrates ethical provisions in all areas of practice.

The holistic registered nurse:

- Uses the *Code of Ethics for Nurses with Interpretive Statements* (ANA, 2001) and *AHNA Position Statement on Holistic Nursing Ethics* to guide practice and articulate the moral foundation of holistic nursing.
- Advocates for the rights of vulnerable, repressed, or underserved populations:

The holistic advanced practice registered nurse:

- Actively contributes to creating an ecosystem that supports well-being for all life.

Standard 13: RESEARCH: The holistic registered nurse integrates research into practice.

The holistic registered nurse:

- Uses the best available evidence, including theories and research findings, to guide practice decisions.
- Actively and ethically participates in research activities related to holistic health at various levels appropriate to the holistic nurse's level of education and position.

The holistic advanced practice registered nurse:

- Contributes to nursing knowledge by conducting or synthesizing research that discovers, examines, and evaluates knowledge, theories, philosophies, context, criteria, and creative approaches to improve holistic health care practice.
- Formally disseminates research findings through activities such as presentations, publications, consultations, and journal clubs for a variety of audiences including nursing, other disciplines, and the public to improve holistic care and further develop the foundation and practice of holistic nursing.

Standard 14: RESOURCE USE: The holistic registered nurse considers factors related to safety, effectiveness, cost, and impact on practice in the planning and delivery of nursing services.

The holistic registered nurse:

- Assists the person, family, and significant others or caregivers as appropriate in identifying and securing appropriate and available services to address health-related needs.
- Identifies discriminatory health care practices as they impact the person and engages in effective nondiscriminatory practices.

The holistic advanced practice registered nurse:

- Uses organizational and community resources to formulate multidisciplinary or interdisciplinary plans of care.

Standard 15: LEADERSHIP: The holistic registered nurse provides leadership in the professional practice setting and the profession.

The holistic registered nurse:

- Displays the ability to define a clear vision, the associated goals, and a plan to implement and measure progress toward holistic health care.
- Promotes advancement of the profession through participation in professional organizations and focusing on strategies that bring unity and healing to the nursing profession.

The holistic advanced practice registered nurse:

- Works to influence decision-making bodies to improve holistic, integrated care.
- Articulates the ideas underpinning holistic nursing philosophy, places these ideas in an historical, philosophical, and scientific context while projecting future trends in thinking.

Appendix 2

The foundation of *Holistic Nursing: Scope and Standards of Practice* (2007) is based on the works of a number of individuals and documents of AHNA including:

American Holistic Nurses Association. AHNA standards of holistic nursing practice. Flagstaff, AZ: Author; 2004.

American Holistic Nurses Association. AHNA standards of advanced holistic nursing practice for graduate prepared nurses. Flagstaff, AZ: Author; revised, 2005.

American Holistic Nurses Association. Description of holistic nursing. Flagstaff, AZ: Author; 1998.

American Holistic Nurses Association. AHNA position statement on the role of nurses in the practice of complementary and alternative therapies. Flagstaff, AZ: Author; reapproved, 2007.

American Holistic Nurses Association. AHNA position statement on nursing research and scholarship. Flagstaff, AZ: Author; updated, 2007.

American Holistic Nurses Association. AHNA position statement on holistic nursing ethics. Flagstaff, AZ: Author; reapproved, 2007.

American Holistic Nurses Association. AHNA position statement on the nursing shortage. Flagstaff, AZ: Author; undated.

Dossey B, editor. Core curriculum for holistic nursing. Gaithersburg, MD: Aspen; 1997.

Dossey B, Keagan L, Guzzetta C. Holistic nursing, a handbook for practice. 4th edition. Gaithersburg, MD: Aspen; 2005.

Frisch N, Dossey B, Guzzette C, et al. AHNA standards of holistic nursing practice with guidelines for caring and healing. Gaithersburg, MD: Aspen; 2000.

Mariano C. An Overview of Holistic Nursing. Imprint 2005;52(2): 1148–52.

Mariano C. Advanced practice in holistic nursing. In: Mezey M, McGivern D, Sullivan-Marx E, editors. Nurse Practitioners Evolution of Advanced Practice. 4th edition. New York: Springer Publishing Company; 2003.

References

[1] American Holistic Nurses Association. AHNA standards of holistic nursing practice. Flagstaff (AZ): American Holistic Nurses Association; revised, 2005.

[2] American Holistic Nurses Association. AHNA standards of advanced holistic nursing practice for graduate prepared nurses. Flagstaff (AZ): American Holistic Nurses Association; revised, 2005.

[3] American Nurses Association. Nursing: scope and standards of practice. Washington, DC: American Nurses Association; 2004.

[4] American Nurses Association. Recognition of a nursing specialty, approval of a specialty nursing scope of practice statement and acknowledgement of specialty nursing standards of practice. Washington, DC: American Nurses Association; 2005.

[5] Mariano C. Proposal for recognition of holistic nursing as a specialty. New York (NY): author; 2006.

[6] American Nurses Association, American Holistic Nurses Association. Holistic nursing: Scope and standards of practice. Washington, DC; 2007, in press.

[7] American Holistic Nurses Association. Description of holistic nursing. Flagstaff (AZ): American Holistic Nurses Association; 1998.

[8] U.S. Department of Health and Human Services. Patient's bill of rights in Medicare and Medicaid. 1999. Available at: www.hhs.gov/news/press/1999pres/990412.html.

[9] American Nurses Association. Code of ethics for nursing with interpretive statements. Washington, DC: American Nurses Association; 2001.

[10] American Holistic Nurses Association. American holistic nurses association position statement on holistic ethics. Flagstaff (AZ): American Holistic Nurses Association; reapproved, 2007.

[11] Dossey B, et al. Evolving a blueprint for certification: Inventory of professional activities and knowledge of a holistic nurse. J Holist Nurs 1998;16(1):33–56.

[12] Watson J. Caring science as sacred science. Philadelphia (PA): FA Davis; 2005. p. 33.

ELSEVIER
SAUNDERS

NURSING
CLINICS
OF NORTH AMERICA

Nurs Clin N Am 42 (2007) 189–212

Legal Parameters of Alternative-Complementary Modalities in Nursing Practice

Sharon Radzyminski, PhD, JD, RN

*School of Nursing, College of Education and Human Services,
Cleveland State University, 2121 Euclid Avenue, Cleveland, OH 44115, USA*

The medical model is the legal "gold standard" by which professional health care practice is recognized and regulated in the United States. Conventional medicine (or biomedicine, as it is often referred to) has dominated health care services in this country for more than a century. Consumer satisfaction with conventional medical practices is circular as opinions shift from almost a God-like adoration with unquestioning obedience to suspicion, criticism, and demand for alternative approaches from health care and alternative care providers. Many of the alternative approaches sought are those that focus on the "whole person" and include elements related to the emotional, mental, environmental, nutritional, cultural, behavioral, and spiritual elements of health. Nurses have traditionally included many of these aspects in their delivery of health care to clients. In the past few decades, nurses have begun to use herbal therapies, massage, aromatherapy, music therapy, guided imagery, meditation, stress management, and spirituality as part of their professional practice. As the demand for alternative therapies increases, questions of liability arise regarding the specific services provided, credibility of those delivering them, and legal boundaries created as multiple professions overlap in providing care for clients. As nurses add these approaches to their professional practice, they need to take into consideration the legal consequences that may accompany these care modalities.

The legal implications for providing complementary or alternative therapies for clients are similar to those associated with standard care. Questions the nurse has to consider include whether the therapy is within his or her scope of practice, whether the therapy overlaps with another profession's

E-mail address: s.radzyminski@csuohio.edu

scope of practice, whether the therapy requires additional education or credentialing, and whether the therapy constitutes enough risk to the client to support a claim of professional negligence or malpractice. To date, litigation specifically against nurses offering alternative therapies has been minimal in comparison to standard care modalities [1]. This, however, may change as various practitioners compete for the same patient population and clients access more alternative treatments for health care problems.

Are complementary and alternative medicine therapies the practice of medicine?

Complementary and alternative therapies are commonly referred to as complementary and alternative medicine (CAM). The name infers that these care modalities are under the auspice of medicine. A common definition used for alternative medicine is that it is medical interventions not taught widely at US medical schools or generally available at US hospitals [1]. As the definition implies, these are "medical" interventions that, although not routinely taught in Western medical schools, are still considered the practice of medicine. The term *alternative* is legally puzzling, however. Alternative suggests that something outside the practice of medicine is available as a substitute that is capable of achieving similar health outcomes. It has been suggested that the terminology should be *alternative "to" medicine* [2], which places these care modalities in a professional arena apart from medical practice. Medicine has also argued that there is no such thing as alternative medicine and that there is only "scientifically proven evidence-based medicine supported by solid data or unproven medicine, for which scientific evidence is lacking" [3]. It makes no difference if it is Eastern or Western in origin or if the philosophic underpinnings involve mind-body integration or genetic manipulation; if the therapy is implemented to target a disease or health condition of a patient, it is the practice of medicine [3]. It remains to be seen which CAM therapies are legally defensible outside the practice of medicine.

One of the first legal issues that presents itself is whether a nurse who offers CAM to clients is practicing medicine without a license. Because licensure is covered under individual state law, the nurse would have to become familiar with the applicable practice acts because they tend to be different between states. If the practice is not specifically covered in the state statute, the legal analysis would include whether there is sufficient evidence to support a claim that the care provided is within the realm of nursing and not that of medicine or other related professions. Sufficient evidence includes but is not limited to historical provision of the care modality, inclusion of the care modality in accredited educational and training programs, recognition of the therapy in professional journals, support by recognized professional organizations, and research conducted by the profession in relation to the care modality. It would therefore be important to begin the evaluation with the historical roots and regulation of CAM practice in relation to the various professions.

Historical provision of complementary and alternative medicine

Complementary and alternative therapies have existed ever since there were accepted standards of professional practice in health care. Medicine is the first profession to identify the use of many of these therapies but has shifted its focus on several occasions. A humorous poem, *A History of Medicine*, by an unknown author depicts this concept rather well [4]:

2000 BC—"Here, eat this root."
1000 AD—"The root is heathen. Say this prayer."
1850 AD—"That prayer is superstitious. Drink this potion."
1940 AD—"That potion is snake oil. Swallow this pill."
1985 AD—"That pill is ineffective. Take this antibiotic."
2000 AD—"That antibiotic doesn't work anymore. Here, eat this root."

The reason for the shift is clear—the current standard of care is ineffective in meeting consumer needs and clients seek alternatives to the standards in an effort to improve their health and well-being. Each time the consumer becomes dissatisfied, the physician falls from grace until a more effective standard can be implemented and restore the physician as the favored practitioner. During this cycle, old standards are replaced with new therapies and the old may become complementary to the new or discarded altogether. If the old standard had therapeutic value, the surfacing of alternative practitioners and their attempts to take ownership of the service are now considered an alternative to the accepted standard. The likelihood of the alternative therapy eventually being retained by the domain of medicine depends on the success rate of the therapy, the acceptance of the therapy by the consumer, the complexity and skill required to provide the therapy, the risk involved, the need for regulation of the therapy, the ability of the therapy to generate financial gain, and the interest of the medical profession in providing the service.

Unfortunately, for the well-educated and skilled alternative health providers of today, previous practitioners outside the mainstream of "official" medicine have a somewhat checkered past. Herbalists, spiritual healers, psychics, magnetic healers, and the like were prolific a century ago in the United States [5]. Most of these individuals had little or no training, no regulation of their practice, and no quality standards by which to be evaluated. Consequently, many patients were seriously harmed, and their practice was labeled as "quackery" [5]. Physicians at the time were not without similar criticism because their skills were typically acquired by undergoing apprenticeships. Because there were no organized schools of medicine, the new practitioner espoused the teaching of his master and this created great rivalry between the various groups of physicians trained by different mentors advocating differing theories of practice. Physician from similar backgrounds and mentors formed "medical societies" to consolidate power and control in their way of thinking and petitioned state legislatures to establish a board that had the authority to examine and license practitioners and prevent anyone who did not conform to their point of view from practicing [6]. By the mid-1800s, all states had their own medical societies that had the authority to grant a license to practice medicine. In the beginning, these licensure laws were rarely enforced and the only penalty for practicing without a license was the inability to sue the patient for unpaid fees. As the societies battled one another over correct standards of practice, schools of medicine were established that also claimed they were qualified to license graduates in the practice of medicine. The legislature of most states allowed the dual licensing system; by 1900, 400 medical schools were founded in the United States. Medical school licensure became popular as students tried to avoid the politics generated by the medical societies. Most of these schools, however, had no affiliation with universities and taught their students such therapies as bloodletting, blistering, and purging. Eventually, there was a public outcry against such practices, and other philosophies of medicine became popular, including thomsonism, which promoted healing through the use of botanical preparations, and homeopathy, which based practice on the belief that what causes disease in a healthy person cures the disease in a sick person. As these forms of medicine became popular, regular physicians banned together to form the American Medical Association (AMA) [7]. The goal of the association was to improve medical education, develop a curriculum based on scientific rigor, and protect the profession against charlatans [7]. Their first goals produced scientific medicine that eliminated such practices as bloodletting and introduced such practices as use of sterile technique in surgery. The latter goal resulted in all "irregular practitioners," such as homeopaths, being expelled from the medical societies and enaction of rules that disallowed any AMA member from consulting with, speaking to, or signing any diploma of a graduate of a mainstream medical school who indicated that he or she supported the practice of "irregular medicine" [8]. Scientific discoveries that resulted in better patient outcomes and the elimination of competitive philosophies of medicine made the AMA the sole voice for the profession of medicine by the early 1900s. By 1910, evaluation of the current medical schools indicated that they needed to be housed in universities engaged in research with regular faculty instead of private physician mentors. Public opinion also began to shift in favor of mainstream medicine as advances in science and technology paved the way for improved patient outcomes, especially in the areas of anesthesia, surgery, and pain control. Because trauma remained a major reason for seeking medical care, homeopathic medicine could not compete with trained surgeons using general anesthesia. State licensing boards increasingly relied on the AMA's recommendations as to whether to honor a school's diploma and eventually failed to license any graduates of institutions not supported by the AMA. By 1913, all homeopathic or alternative schools of medicine had closed or converted to the curriculum approved by the AMA. Physicians made it clear that complementary or alternative therapies were not accepted as the practice of medicine [8].

This turbulent time in medicine's history is also the century when other health professions emerged and attempted to set practice boundaries separate from or complementary to the practice of medicine. Nursing emerged in the latter part of the nineteenth century with its own philosophy and research base. Before the 1800s, nursing was not considered an intellectual endeavor but a service provided by religious orders or reserved for the immoral, drunken, and illiterate women of the day or prostitutes. Duties consisted mainly of housework and cleaning or simple procedures, such as bloodletting or purging [9].

In 1869, Florence Nightingale founded the Nightingale School Home for Nurses at Saint Thomas Hospital in London, thereby issuing nurses into the arena of trained health professionals available for public use [10]. Nursing was re-established with a distinct philosophy, practice boundaries, educational requirements, and body of knowledge based on research. According to Nightingale [11], nurses were to "put patients in the best condition for nature to act upon him." Nursing practice was based on statistical and epidemiologic data in identified areas, such as ventilation, sensory stimulation, nutrition and feeding, rest and activity, hygiene, patient education, and patient assessment. Nursing's identified areas of practice evolved around nurturing, healing, restoration of health, and support services. Because medicine concentrated on episodic care, surgical skill, and diagnostic techniques, nurses, who practiced mainly in the home, became skilled experts in supportive and rehabilitative therapies. Complementary and noninvasive alternative therapies were clearly housed in the profession of nursing and considered outside the realm of medicine. If history ended here, certain CAM modalities would probably simply be referred to as "nursing practice." This, however, changed as health care delivery advanced in the twentieth century. Boundaries became blurred when both professions began to offer services primarily within institutional settings to the same patient population. The skills of research so stressed by Nightingale were lost as nursing education shifted its emphasis to skill acquisition to keep pace with medical advances. Skills, such as measuring patient blood pressures or administering medications, once only performed by physicians, became part of nursing services as physicians abandoned these practices for those requiring newer skills and higher levels of education. Physicians maintained that these activities remained the practice of medicine but allowed specially trained or educated nurses to provide these "advanced practice" procedures or therapies so long as they performed them under the control and supervision of a physician. This process was not unique to medicine, however. As nurses aligned their practice closer and closer to medicine, other health professions emerged to take over the care delivery practices once claimed by nursing. Nursing, unlike medicine, however, rarely lobbied the legislature to include these individuals under nurse practice acts and were content to share practice with other professions, such as respiratory therapy or dieticians. Practice issues similar to those seen earlier between the various medical societies began to surface as nursing struggled to maintain a separate professional identity. The ability to separate medicine and nursing became increasingly difficult as nursing began to pattern its health care delivery practices after the medical model. Professional licensure regulations were faced with providing two types of guidelines. The first was the right to practice the given profession, and the second was the right to practice another profession under certain regulated and controlled circumstances. In the former, the individual is responsible for his or her own professional practice. In the latter, responsibility for practice is jointly shared and regulation and guidelines for practice are set by the profession under which the licensee is practicing. This is an important distinction when a decision has to be made on whether an individual is practicing a profession without a license; practicing another profession under that profession's consent, guidance, and supervision; the degree of duty the individual has toward the client; and the standards to which the individual is held.

Licensure

The right to practice a health care profession is controlled by the regulatory authority of the state under its police power [12]. Police power is part of state sovereignty and refers to its supreme and absolute powers. It is the public authority that sets the limits under which its citizens may act. In the exercise of its "police power," a state has the authority to regulate, restrain, or prohibit that which is harmful to the public welfare, even though the regulation, restraint, or prohibition might interfere with an individual's liberty or property [13]. This is important, because every citizen has a constitutional right to engage in any legitimate occupation, including the health professions, under the Fourteenth Amendment [14]. When health professionals assert their right to practice, however, they face the state's authority to protect its citizens' health, safety, and welfare. In these situations, the state is the absolute power, for which there is no appeal. Therefore, anyone licensed by the state to practice a profession is bound by the language of the practice statute. When nurses seek to add alternative or complementary therapies to their professional practice, they must do so in accordance with their state's nurse practice act and be certain that the practice has not been delineated to another profession's practice.

Professional practice acts establish the codes of conduct for the licensees and establish boards to regulate educational and practice requirements as well as to discipline those who violate the act. Many prohibit the delivery of certain health care services by unlicensed persons as in medicine. In the pursuit as to whether the therapy in question lies within the nurse practice act, one must first identify the therapy in question. The National Institutes of Health (NIH) classify CAM practices into seven subsets [15]:

1. Mind-body interventions (psychotherapy, support groups, meditation, guided imagery, hypnosis, biofeedback, yoga, dance therapy, music therapy, art therapy, prayer, and mental healing)
2. Bioelectromagnetic applications in medicine (nonthermal non-ionizing electromagnetic fields, nerve stimulation, neuroacupuncture, immune system stimulation, and neuroendocrine modulations)
3. Alternative systems of medical practice (traditional oriental medicine, acupuncture, Ayurveda, homeopathic medicine, anthroposophically extended medicine, and Native American medicine)
4. Manual healing methods (osteopathic medicine, chiropractic science, massage therapy, and biofield therapeutics)
5. Pharmacologic and biologic treatments (antineoplastins, cartilage products, ethylenediaminetetraacetic acid [EDTA] chelation therapy, and immunoaugmentative therapy)
6. Herbal medicine (Chinese herbal medicines, Ayurvedic herbal medicines, and Native American herbal medicines)
7. Diet and nutrition (vitamin and nutritional supplements, megavitamin therapy, Gerson therapy, Kelly regimen, macrobiotics, Livingston/Wheeler regimen, Wigmore treatment, Ornish diet, and diets from all other cultures)

As one can see, CAM therapies may cross multiple professional boundaries, and it is beyond the scope of this article to investigate each practice. Individuals should be alert that many of these therapies are regulated by state practice acts and require a license to perform. Chiropractic, massage therapy, acupuncture, and naturopathy are four of the most commonly licensed modalities. Although nurses seldom engage in acupuncture and chiropractic science, they should be aware of what might be covered in other professional practice acts. For example naturopathy emphasizes preventative and lifestyle health measures, including nutrition. Naturopaths use herbal medicine, vitamins, and mineral supplements to support and strengthen body systems and restore balance. Although nutritional counseling is generally accepted as part of the nurse practice act, herbal counseling may be considered the practice of naturopathy in some states [16].

Licensure is the privilege of the individual states and may be different from one to another. All 50 states have medical and nursing practice acts and various occupational licensures. Licensure creates a minimum level of professional competence, exerts some degree of quality control, and prevents other professionals from gaining control over the licensed profession. Professional licensing has three options. Mandatory licensure is the highest level and prohibits all unlicensed providers from providing the services. The

most common example is medicine and all who practice within the parameters of medicine (eg, dentists, podiatrists, veterinarians, osteopaths, phar-
macists) as well as those directly supervised by medicine (eg, physician
assistants, respiratory therapists) [17]. Title licensure makes a demonstrable
level of skill or training mandatory for those who claim a particular occupational title. Uncertified providers cannot be charged with unlawful practice
so long as they do not use the statutory-defined title. This is common among
psychology licensing statutes, which allow many professionals to practice
psychology; however, only a licensed psychologist may use the title "psychologist" [5]. The third type of licensure is registration, in which the individual must simply register with the state to practice [5]. Massage therapy is
a common example, although some states now have mandatory massage
therapy licensure. Nurses should contact their state boards of nursing to inquire about the existence and level of professional practice statutes before
implementing any type of alternative therapies.

To determine whether any given therapy in question falls within the parameters of a legally identified profession, a careful reading of the licensure
statue is required. In relation to the practice of medicine, most states include
language related to diagnosing, preventing, treating, and curing disease; performing surgery; and using, administering, or prescribing drugs or medicinal
preparations. These statutes are often vague and meant to encompass a wide
array of health care services. If taken literally, almost no known therapy
falls outside the practice of medicine. Thereby, it could be argued that unless
stated otherwise, all CAM therapies are within the practice of medicine. If,
however, it can be shown that the therapy in question is contained within
the independent practice of another profession, the therapy can be provided
by those licensed professionals as well. The question then becomes whether
there are areas of practice contained within the nurse practice act that the
nurse can perform independently without the consent or supervision of
a physician. If so, it is the practice of nursing.

By 1923, all states had enacted nurse licensure laws. These early laws,
however, merely regulated the title "registered nurse" rather than the practice of nursing. These laws were strictly title statutes. Anyone could perform
the duties of a nurse, but only those who were licensed could call themselves
a registered nurse. In 1938, New York became the first state to elevate its
nurse practice act to mandatory status. It attempted to define nursing practice and prohibited unlicensed persons from engaging in nursing practice.
This allowed registered nurses to perform tasks and make judgments independent of physician supervision. These "tasks" were carefully identified,
and most state statutes contained language that prohibited nursing from engaging in diagnosis and treatment. *Treatment* became a defining term in the
limitation of nursing practice. If nurses were not allowed to treat a patient
under their own professional license, what activities or tasks were they actually permitted to do? Even basic activities, such as ambulating a patient,
changing surgical dressings, or the method of bathing a patient, had to be

"ordered" by a physician. Nursing practice was interpreted as performing the duties nurses were directed to do. For example, the best and most efficient way to feed a patient was within the practice of nursing, but the decision of which diet to choose had to be ordered by the physician. Unfortunately for the nurse, he or she could not initiate the feeding until he or she knew what to feed, how much, and how often. Nursing was not defined as a profession with its own phenomena of interest, practice boundaries, or body of knowledge but, rather, as individuals skilled to perform tasks and procedures under the direction of a physician. Nurses attempted to change this image and developed the "nursing process" in the 1950s to demonstrate nurses' ability to assess, evaluate, and initiate treatment as independent practitioners.

In 1971, Idaho was the first state to amend its nurse practice act to qualify the statutory prohibitions related to diagnosis and treatment by allowing the state boards of medicine and nursing jointly to authorize regulations recognizing independent nursing practice [18]. New York followed, amending its practice act in 1972 by defining "diagnosis" as the "identification of and discrimination between physical and psychosocial signs and symptoms essential to the effective execution and management of a nursing regimen. Such diagnostic privilege is distinct from a medical diagnosis [19]." The ability of organized nursing to define nursing practice outside the medical model was instrumental in establishing independence from the medical profession and reducing the risk of nurses being charged with the unauthorized practice of medicine. Many current nurse practice acts include the terms *diagnosis* and *treatment* as part of the language used to describe nursing practice. For example, Florida defines the practice of nursing as "the observation, assessment, nursing diagnosis, planning, intervention, and evaluation, health teaching and counseling of the ill, injured, or infirm; and the promotion of wellness, maintenance of health, and prevention of illness of others" [20]. The statute goes on to define nursing diagnosis as the "observation and evaluation of physical or mental behaviors, signs and symptoms of illness, and reactions to treatment and the determination of whether such conditions, signs, symptoms, and reactions represent a deviation from health status" [20]. Nursing treatment is defined as the "establishment and implementation of a nursing regimen, care and comfort of individuals, the prevention of illness, and the education, restoration and maintenance of health" [20]. Oregon states that the practice of nursing "means diagnosing and treating human responses to actual or potential health problems through such services as identification thereof, health teaching, health counseling and providing care supportive to or restorative of life and well-being including the performance of such additional services requiring education and training which are recognized by the nursing profession as proper to be performed by a licensed nurse ..." [21]. Statutes like these are significant in several ways. First, there is a deliberate attempt to use the terms *diagnosis* and *treatment* in the definition of the profession. This is a clear indication of the state's acknowledgment that diagnosis and treatment do not exclusively rest in the domain of medicine. Second, the definitions do not include restrictions, such as "under the direction or supervision of a physician." The practice of nursing, as defined, refers to the independent scope of professional practice.

Other states are more restrictive. Texas claims that professional nursing is the "performance of an act that requires substantial specialized judgment and skill, the proper performance of which is based on knowledge and application of the principles of biological, physical, and social science as acquired by a completed course in an approved school of professional nursing. The term does not include acts of medical diagnosis or the prescription of therapeutic or corrective measures" [22]. Absent is the complete lack of the use of such terms as *diagnosis* or *treatment*, except in the disclaimer. Also, nursing is defined as merely the "performance of an act" that is learned in an approved school of nursing. According to the Texas statute, a nurse would be outside the nurse practice act if he or she attempted to provide care that was not learned as part of the nursing school curriculum or initiated professional care based on cognitive or intellectual processes. The Texas statute further defines acts to include the observation, assessment, intervention, evaluation, rehabilitation, care, counsel, and health teachings of the ill, injured, or infirmed [22]. This insinuates that a nurse can independently initiate interventions based on evaluation of observations or assessments. Taken in context with the professional definition, these interventions are restricted to those learned in nursing schools and the initiation of such cannot be construed as the prescription of therapeutic or corrective measures. Neither prescription nor therapeutic or corrective measures are defined by the nurse practice act, which may place these activities within the practice of medicine in the state of Texas.

Nurse practice acts still remain open to interpretation, however, regardless of specific language used. Although nursing treatments are recognized in Florida as within the boundaries of professional nursing practice, there remain questions about what is included, for example, in the care and comfort of individuals or the prevention of illness. Taken as written, it could be argued that almost any treatment, including CAM, could be construed as providing care or comfort or preventing illness. The key, of course, is that it must be, by definition, a nursing treatment.

In addition to professional practice acts, a few states also have general provisions specifically for complementary or alternative health care therapies. Florida statute §456.41 states that a health care practitioner "may in his or her discretion and without restriction, recommend any mode of treatment that is, in his or her best judgment, in the best interests of the patient, including complementary or alternative health care treatments, in accordance with the provisions of his or her license" [20]. This language is typical of state statues and is aimed to shield the care provider against allegations of "unprofessional conduct" based on deviations from the accepted and prevailing practice of the profession as held by the state board of professional practice. These statutes typically do not address issues related to whether a particular therapy is within the scope of practice of a particular profession.

State boards of nursing are a source for interpreting licensure laws and provide guidance to nurses who wish to incorporate these therapies into their professional practice. Many boards have a formal policy, positions, or specific language related to alternative or complementary therapies available. The Arizona Board of Nursing was one of the first to issue a formal advisory opinion statement in 1991, which was quickly followed by the Kentucky, Massachusetts, and Pennsylvania Boards of Nursing. Most statements refer to the practice of energy-based modalities, such as healing touch, therapeutic touch, and massage therapies. These modalities are recognized to be within the scope of practice of a professional nurse in 25 states and are under discussion in an additional 7 states [23].

This leads to the second part of the legal analysis. If it can be shown that the therapy in question is a treatment and treatments are within the scope of practice in the state's licensure statute, it must then be analyzed to determine if it is a nursing treatment. To do this, evidence must be presented that the modality in question is included in accredited educational and training programs, the modality is supported by recognized professional organizations, or that research is being conducted by the profession in relation to the care modality.

Are complementary and alternative therapies included in educational curricula?

Certain CAM therapies, such as chiropractic science, acupuncture, homeopathic medicine, and naturopathy, are clearly regulated in some states and are subject to licensure laws. With other therapies, however, there is no clear delineation that inclusion of the therapy in practice is within the boundaries of any one specific profession by history or through licensure. If licensure laws are vague but do not expressly prohibit the practice, courts frequently look at professional standards and education to provide evidence that the therapy is within an individual's scope of practice [5].

It has been reported that more than 60% of medical schools in the United States now teach alternative medical practices [24] as separate courses or special topics in required courses. Several prestigious medical schools, such as the Columbia College of Physicians and Surgeons and University of California at San Francisco, have developed specific centers for the study and practice of integrative medicine. The Group for Educational Affairs of the Association of American Medical Colleges created a special interest category specifically aimed at introducing CAM therapies into medical school curricula [25]. Once considered the work of charlatans, medical schools are now introducing students to a broad range of modalities, such as massage therapy, acupuncture, traditional oriental medicine, nutritional and herbal medicine, folk medicine, spirituality, and mind-body therapies.

Nursing curricula have been much less responsive. With few exceptions, traditional nursing education in undergraduate and graduate nursing programs continues to follow the medical model. Advanced practice in nursing has concentrated on educating practitioners to become skilled in assessment and procedures that were once within the scope of medical practice. There are some noted exceptions, however. The University of Minnesota and Rush University College of Nursing have embraced holistic nursing as their theoretic framework and regularly include CAM components in their curricula. The University of California at San Francisco's Nurse Practitioner Program has incorporated CAM through its Integrated Complementary Healing Program [26]. Prominent nurse theorists, such as Roy, use concepts like as focal, contextual, and residual stimulation as a basis for nursing interventions. Aromatherapy and music therapy are among the nursing interventions supported by Roy's theory of adaptation [27]. Watson [28], another noted nurse theorist, portrays nursing as a caring-healing paradigm with many complementary or alternative therapies as relevant to her care-based theoretic framework. In nursing, however, there is no universally accepted theoretic framework under which nursing curricula are organized, such that the teaching of CAM is inconsistent. There is agreement in the profession, however, that all accepted theories take into the account the whole person [29] and address the physical, mental, emotional, and spiritual dimensions of care. As such, the theoretic foundation of nursing practice is seen as holistic in nature. The American Association of Colleges of Nursing (AACN) has attempted to acknowledge the presence of CAM as part of professional nursing practice by including CAM in its essentials document for baccalaureate and master's education [30].

The development of nursing taxonomies has also been helpful for providing frameworks for naming and documenting the phenomena of nursing practice. The North American Nursing Diagnosis Association (NANDA) classification of nursing diagnoses lists more than 150 recognized nursing diagnoses organized according to domains based on health patterns [31]. In addition the Nursing Interventions Classification (NIC) [32] and the Nursing Outcomes Classification (NOC) [33] list nursing activities that have been identified by nurses as actions they perform in direct care activities that are sensitive to nursing interventions. These documentation systems are valuable in the establishment of a therapy as a nursing treatment or nursing action as referred to in nurse practice acts. Unfortunately, nurses do not always document their assessments or interventions in accordance with the established taxonomies, which makes the legal analysis of their actions more challenging.

Of great concern is that nurses are being taught these therapies by non-nurses and outside accredited educational programs. This places the therapy outside the context of professional nursing and makes it difficult to defend as a treatment within the boundaries of nurse practice acts.

Professional associations

Professional associations are tied to practice issues in that they are often consultants to licensure statutes and liability issues related to scope of practice and standard of care. To have legal influence, the association must be considered a spokesperson for the profession; otherwise, literally hundreds of organizations would need to be recognized. For the association to have legal influence, its mission should be to establish educational requirements for the profession; establish standards of practice; set standards of professional conduct or ethics; promote research in the profession; and promote public recognition of the profession, including influencing public policy [12].

The AMA House of Delegates passed a policy in 1994, which it reaffirmed in 1995, encouraging its members "to become better informed regarding alternative medicine and to participate in appropriate studies" [34]. As of May 2006, the AMA's policy statement on alternative medicine states [35]:

> (1) There is little evidence to confirm the safety or efficacy of most alternative therapies. Much of the information currently known about these therapies makes it clear that many have not been shown to be efficacious. Well-designed, stringently controlled research should be done to evaluate the efficacy of alternative therapies. (2) Physicians should routinely inquire about the use of alternative or unconventional therapy by their patients, and educate themselves and their patients about the state of scientific knowledge with regard to alternative therapy that may be used or contemplated. (3) Patients who choose alternative therapies should be educated as to the hazards that might result from postponing or stopping conventional medical treatment.

The American Nurses Association has no relevant policy but supports the American Holistic Nurses Association as an organization representative of nursing professional practice. Holistic nursing is defined as "all nursing practice that has healing the whole person as its goal" [36]. As part of its defining statement, it claims to be "different from other nursing practice ... and requires the nurse to integrate self-care and self-responsibility into his or her own life and to strive for an awareness of the interconnectedness of individuals to the human and global community" [36]. This statement indicates that professional nursing recognizes that care practices "different" from mainstream modalities remain within the boundaries of professional nursing practice. The association supports nursing interventions and holistic care therapies that are consistent with research findings and other sound evidence, offers certification credentialing to its nurses, and publishes the *Journal of Holistic Nursing*. The association and professional journals provide a vehicle to identify and research care modalities considered by the profession to be part of the practice of nursing. Membership in the association is low, however, in relation to the number of licensed nurses eligible, thereby casting doubt on the general acceptance of these practices by the profession as a whole.

Research and governmental initiatives

The National Center for Complementary and Alternative Medicine (NCCAM) is currently one of the 27 institutes and centers that make up the NIH [15]. Its mission is to explore complementary and healing practices in the context of rigorous science, train CAM researchers, and disseminate authoritative information to the public and professionals [15]. Relatively new, it was established in October 1991 when Congress passed legislation (P.L. 102-170) to fund an Office of Alternative Medicine within the NIH. It funded its first phase III clinical trial in 1997 on St. John's wort for depression with the National Institute of Mental Health and the NIH Office of Dietary Supplements. It was officially established as the NCCAM in 1998 under Title VI, Section 601 of the Omnibus Appropriations Act. The NCAMM Director was thereby vested with broad decision-making authority concerning financial and administrative management and fiscal and review responsibility for grants and contracts. In June 2002, the NCCAM launched its first intramural study on the use of electracupuncture to treat chemotherapy-induced nausea. To date, the NCCAM has funded approximately 1200 research projects at scientific institutions and provides an information clearinghouse, fact sheets, a Distinguished Lecture series, continuing medical education programs, and publication databases [15].

There is no equivalent center in the National Institute of Nursing Research, but because the NCAAM's mission is to explore complementary and alternative healing practices and not medicine, it encompasses all CAM practitioners. Funded research has been largely medical in nature, however. There have been some instances of funded research for CAM therapies awarded to nursing. The University of California at San Francisco does have a 3-year federal government grant to sustain its Integrated Complementary Healing Program [26].

In March 2000, President Clinton signed Executive Order 13.147 establishing the White House Commission on Complementary and Alternative Medicine to "address education and training of health care practitioners in CAM, coordinate research to increase knowledge about CAM products, provide reliable and useful information on CAM to health professions, and provide guidance on the appropriate access to and delivery of CAM" [37]. The Commission's final report issued in March 2002 urged funding of demonstration projects to identify the best models for integrating CAM and conventional medicine. Suggested models included conventional and

CAM practitioners working side-by-side as equals and CAM practitioners working independently but under a physician's supervision [38]. Notably missing was the suggestion that professional CAM practitioners outside the profession of medicine would be recognized as independent providers of care under their own professional license. The Commission further urged that CAM practitioner training should include basic biomedical language, medical record maintenance, health care law, referral practices and how to collaborate with conventional providers [39].

Complementary and alternative medicine modalities within nursing's scope of practice

Within the categories of CAM-recognized modalities, it could be argued that many are within the scope of practice for nursing. Some of the commonly identified therapies include herbal therapy, aromatherapy, massage, music therapy, guided imagery, meditation, therapeutic touch, and stress management. Although these therapies may be recognized as nursing treatments in some states, nurses who perform them should be aware of issues that may be associated with the practices.

Herbal therapy

Herbs, vitamins, minerals, amino acids, and similar substances are classified as dietary supplements, and thereby a subcategory of food. The Dietary Supplement Health and Education Act of 1994 (DSHEA) allows these products to be marketed without receiving US Food and Drug Administration (FDA) approval, and they are not considered medications [40]. This distinction may release nurses from many nurse practice act restrictions that place administration of medications under the supervision of a physician. This is not always true, however. Courts sometimes err on the side of finding scope-of-practice violations to be extremely broad. For example, health care professionals have been charged with the unlawful practice of medicine for recommending dietary supplements to patients, even though these products are available in retail stores [41]. If nurses recommend, educate, or counsel patients on herbal therapies, they have to show evidence of their acquisition of knowledge and skill level. Herbal therapy is not routinely taught as part of nursing curricula, except occasionally as an elective or as a module within a nutrition or pharmacology course. This is not sufficient training for nurses to be able to claim it is a nursing treatment within nursing's scope of practice. Nurses engaging in this type of therapy should also inquire as to whether there are state regulations surrounding this practice and whether advanced education or credentialing is required. Because many herbs and other dietary supplements are untested, the nurse is also liable for professional negligence if the therapy proves harmful. Within a nurse's scope of practice, however, is the need for nursing to collect a history of herbal use by patients as part of patient assessment data.

Massage

Backrubs have been recognized as a nursing treatment for as long as nursing has been recognized as a profession. Simple massage, such as back-rubs used to improve patient comfort, is considered an independent nursing intervention. Therapeutic massage, however, is classified as a distinct occupation in 27 states and requires practitioners to be licensed before they can provide this therapy [5].

Aromatherapy

Aromatherapy is the therapeutic use of essential oils to treat various health-related problems. It has a strong historical base in nursing practice and was taught in all the original Nightingale schools [10]. Since the mid-1900s, however, the use of essential oils in nursing practice has not routinely been incorporated in nursing curricula. The nurse would need to show evidence of knowledge acquisition similar to those using herbal therapy. Because many essential oils are not well tested and the patient typically inhales these substances, the nurse is at risk for negligence or unprofessional behavior if the patient has an unfavorable outcome. Historical use or common use in other societies is not an adequate defense for malpractice.

Guided imagery or meditation

Guided imagery uses mental images and exercises to help the mind "see" positive or desired outcomes to improve health and well-being. It is noninvasive, and thereby carries a low risk of liability. There remains the question, however, as to whether this therapy is part of nursing education or a technique learned outside the profession.

Therapeutic touch

The concept of therapeutic touch is derived from the ancient practice of "laying on the hands," and various versions of this therapy have been practiced since the time of Hippocrates. It was reintroduced to nursing by Dolores Krieger in 1975. Through therapeutic touch, the practitioner modulates the flow of human energy through the use of hands [42]. It may include some physical contact, but it is not a requirement for assessment and treatment, and therefore carries a low risk of liability. Although therapeutic touch is not routinely taught as part of most nursing curricula, a large percentage of research studies using the therapy are conducted in reference to nursing phenomena by nurse researchers. Research findings are commonly reported in professional nursing journals. In relation to all CAM therapies, therapeutic touch has the highest probability of being considered nursing practice and is currently recognized in 25 states in their nurse practice acts [23]. This is not the case with Reiki, a similar modality that uses a Japanese technique to promote healing through stress reduction and relaxation. The ability to use Reiki is typically transferred to the student during a Reiki class [43], and it is therefore seldom taught in nursing schools or by professional nurses.

Legal considerations for nurses using complementary and alternative medicine outside professional practice issues

Typically, there is far less patient-initiated litigation involving professionals using CAM therapies than those who comply with the standard of care. Alternative medicine claims account for less than 5% of professional malpractice litigation [1]. It is believed that the lack of basis for suit is related to the largely noninvasive nature of the therapies, which result in less severe injuries. CAM therapies typically require more direct patient contact, and patients are less likely to sue practitioners whom they view as supportive. Nonetheless, CAM therapies can carry significant legal liabilities [1], which are discussed next.

Professional malpractice or negligence

A nurse providing CAM treatments is subject to the same professional standards as with conventional nursing care. In a malpractice claim, it would have to be shown that that the nurse had a duty to the patient, that there was a breach in that duty, and that the patient incurred harm as a direct result of the nurse's actions [44]. Nurses have a duty to provide safe care and to stay current with literature on any therapy they provide. They also have a duty to assess their patients adequately. It is estimated that more than 15 million Americans are taking high-dose vitamins, mineral supplements, or herbal preparations or are participating in some diet regimen in addition to taking prescription drugs, which may adversely affect their health status. Questions related to alternative therapy use should be incorporated in every nurse's patient assessment.

By definition, there must be harm incurred by the patient for a malpractice claim to go forward. Because many CAM therapies, such as guided imagery, therapeutic touch, simple massage, or meditation, carry a low risk of physical injury, malpractice claims have been minimal for these treatments. Therapies that include the ingestion or inhalation of a substance carry greater risk.

Professional discipline

Professional practice acts establish boards that oversee the licensee's conduct and grant authority to the board to induce penalties for any licensee's misconduct. Most boards have the right to sanction members of their own profession that engage in "unprofessional conduct," which includes "departure from" or "failure to conform to" standards of acceptable practice [45]. Although this is usually reserved for those who practice incompetently or negligently, it has been used on occasion for those who practice CAM therapies because such therapies are, by definition, a departure from standard practice. It is important to note that professional discipline does not require that the patient be harmed but only that the practitioner deviate from acceptable and prevailing practice [45]. Some states, such as Florida, have enacted CAM statutes that shield health professionals from professional discipline under certain circumstances.

Recklessness

Professionals are considered reckless if they participate in a practice that they know little about. Although there is anecdotal, historical, and cultural evidence for many alternative therapies, many lack well-designed clinical studies that examine their efficacy and safety. Take, for example, a nurse who provides herbal therapy counseling as an independent practice. If the nurse recommends a dietary supplement that has not been subjected to evidence-based reviews to a patient for a specific condition and sells the patient the product, he or she may be liable not only for malpractice but for recklessness [46]. Nurses should only rely on evidence-based research for information and not on propriety-based research. If the only research available on a product is by the company that produces it, that is not likely to be considered sufficient evidence to refute a malpractice claim.

Informed consent/failure to warn

Informed consent means that the individual possesses all information relevant to determine what is going to be done to his or her own body. Typically, obtaining informed consent rests with the physician, but the informed consent doctrine is applicable to any professional who is providing treatment sanctioned by his or her own professional license. When determining whether proper consent has been obtained, the court investigates whether the provider of the treatment adequately described the condition for which the therapy is recommended, the purpose of the treatment, the expected outcomes, the risks involved, the likelihood of the treatment being effective, and the availability of other potential treatments [47]. In many CAM therapies, including but not limited to dietary supplements, herbal therapy, aromatherapy, and diet therapy, evidence-based research is limited; thus, many of the elements of informed consent are unknown. Nurses should be diligent in making sure their patients are aware that the possibility of unknown risk exists. In addition, if a patient discloses the use of such items as dietary supplements to the nurse and the nurse neither acknowledges nor discourages the practice, the patient may assume that the practice was approved by the nurse. If the patient later experiences harm by the continued use of the supplement that he or she now believes has been approved by the nurse, he or she may have a claim for failure to warn. When a patient discloses his or her participation in alternative therapies that have not been adequately researched, the nurse should provide the patient with that information and record the conversation in the patient care record.

Fraud

Because many CAM therapies are not generally accepted within the biomedical community and products lack FDA approval, providing such treatments is subject to reach under broad antifraud rules [48]. Typically, these claims are not made for noninvasive therapies or treatments not submitted to third-party payers for reimbursement. A claim of fraud could be initiated if the health care provider led the patient to believe that the treatment is effective when there is no definitive evidence to support the claim. Suits have been forthcoming against CAM providers for "malicious distribution of false and misleading information" when patients have based their decision to undergo therapy for health-related problems in lieu of standard care on such information [48]. Because there is limited scientific evidence on many dietary supplements and essential oils, nurses should be careful in how they address these subjects with their patients. Even suggestions that garlic can reduce blood pressure or cinnamon can lower blood glucose levels can be construed as fraud if the patient claims the nurse distributed information that led him or her to believe that the consumption of such products was as effective or as well tested as the standard treatment for such conditions.

Liability as an unlicensed provider

Given that some states allow unlicensed individuals to provide CAM treatments without encroaching on the unlawful practice of medicine, questions arise regarding the liability of the nurse who administers CAM therapies as a lay provider instead of holding himself or herself out as a nurse. In the law of torts, there are two standards for CAM providers: malpractice and ordinary negligence. Malpractice is commonly used for licensed health care professionals, and negligence or breach of contract is used for unlicensed CAM providers. When determining the degree of liability of an individual, courts often evaluate the skill that the practitioner purports to possess and evidence of the practitioner's actual methods, training, and skill [49]. The standard for proving negligence is whether the person used the same degree of reasonable care and skill expected of other practitioners in same or similar circumstances. This standard would therefore be less if the person were a lay practitioner rather than a nurse. The courts are not so easily fooled, however. They would take into consideration the individual's education and training and apply it to a reasonable person standard.

The question would be if a reasonable nurse would offer this therapy and whether the therapy deviates from the "professional standards of skill and care" prevailing among those who offer the treatment as registered nurses.

CAM liability for injuries is usually brought under malpractice claims, but there are other possible causes of action, such as contract law and unfair trade practices. A case in point is when an injured plaintiff claimed that when her physician used CAM techniques along with conventional medical therapy for treatment of her multiples sclerosis, he transformed his practice into an entrepreneurial enterprise, which subjected him to the law of unfair trade practices [50]. The court rejected these arguments, because "entrepreneurial aspects" of practice refer to solicitation of business and billing practices rather than medical treatments. If, however, it could be shown that the treatments were offered in an attempt to solicit business, that might be sufficient to move this case into the realm of unfair trade practices [50].

Contract law is another avenue available to individuals harmed by CAM therapies. If the care provider and the patient meet the legal requirements of a contract, including mutual assent, offer, acceptance, and consideration, an injured patient may claim that the provider's treatments constituted a material breach of a contract term. For example, the patient could allege that the CAM provider failed to perform the solicited treatment in the manner or frequency promised and that this failure resulted in the patient's injury.

Other less used claims include breach of warranty or strict tort liability. Under a warranty claim, a patient would need to establish that the service or treatment provided did not culminate in the promised health outcome. If the CAM treatments consist primarily of goods, such as herbs or essential oils, the Uniform Commercial Code (UCC), which sets forth the rules that control commercial transactions and contracts in all states (except Louisiana), would apply to the breach of warranty action as well.

The doctrine of strict tort liability can be used by any consumer of services against anyone in the chain of product distribution for a defect in a product if that defect is found to make the product unreasonably dangerous to the user of the product. In reference to CAM providers, should an oil, herb, supplement, or any other product used in therapy be found to be harmful and the product was provided by the CAM therapist, the therapist may be liable for the patient's injuries.

Use of the Internet and complementary and alternative medicine therapies

A new and emerging body of law that also applies to CAM practitioners is the area of E-Health. E-Health is the "emerging field in the intersection of medical information, public health, and business, referring to health services and information delivered or enhanced through the Internet and related technologies" [51]. E-Health law would apply to those who offer health information, patient education, or health care marketing over the Internet. If a nurse establishes a Web site and offers services that cross state lines and the nurse does not have a license to practice nursing in the states in which his or her clients are housed, the nurse may be practicing nursing without a license in those states. All states require that a nurse who provides nursing care, which includes patient education or health information, for a patient located in the state must hold a valid license in that state. Therefore, if a patient in Texas receives health information from a nurse in Oklahoma over the Internet, the nurse in Oklahoma is potentially practicing nursing in Texas without a license.

Summary

The law is established to protect the public from dangerous or worthless treatments or therapies and to sanction inappropriate behavior by those who provide them. It is done through licensure laws, food and drug laws, state health care professional boards, tort law (eg, malpractice), and other miscellaneous legal actions. Alternative therapies are, by definition, outside the mainstream standards for accepted care modalities. Whenever a nurse elects to participate in such therapies, the nurse should be aware of the risks involved for his or her own professional practice and the safety of his or her patients.

Health care law regarding CAM is changing. Once hostile to competing therapy, the legal system is recognizing the patient's right to access holistic and integrative care and the practitioner's right to provide it. Medicine, which once routinely disciplined practitioners for participating in alternative care strategies, now includes such language as holism, integrated whole, spiritualism, self-care, nutritional treatment, emotive therapies, massage, and energy healing in its professional literature, medical school curricula, and research agendas. Nursing, which historically based its practice on many of these same principles, has been slower to recognize these elements in its care modalities. It is unlikely that licensure statutes are going to be written clearly identifying overlap of professional services. Boundaries of professional practice are likely to continue to be evaluated based on the profession's education and training of its members, phenomena of interest, research in identified areas and care modalities, reports in the literature, and support by professional organizations.

In addition to issues related to professional practice, safety and efficacy of alternative modalities are likely to continue to be of legal concern. The use of herbs, diet, exercise, essential oils, massage, spirituality, and multiple other therapies has been recognized as components of health for centuries, but many aspects of these therapies are untested or minimally tested. Historically, their value has not been evaluated in light of currently available treatments. If nurses are to incorporate these modalities into their professional practice, they must do so with care. It should be clear that the historical provision of alternative therapies or their routine use in other cultures is not sufficient to sustain a claim of safe practice. Vintage nursing texts are full of recommended therapies that were not in the patient's best interest, and Florence Nightingale herself taught nurses to disregard microorganisms as a cause of disease. Untested care practices should only be administered with adequate informed consent under research conditions. Evidence-based practice should be the goal of every professional nurse.

The profession of nursing needs to take a hard look at its continued support of the medical model for nursing curricula and to take a proactive approach if nurses wish to maintain holistic care under the auspice of professional nursing. If these therapies are to be considered the practice of nursing and not medicine, physical therapy, respiratory therapy, occupational therapy, massage therapy, or any other occupation or profession, nursing needs to address these subjects in curriculum development and professional standards uniformly and provide research to demonstrate the efficacy and safety of these modalities. Nursing is in a unique position to research issues and therapies that explore the interconnections between mind, body, emotions, spirit, and health. Nursing was founded on this premise. Perhaps it is time to reconsider this before these practices legally belong to someone else.

References

[1] Studdert D, Eisenberg D, Miller F, et al. Medical malpractice implications of alternative medicine. JAMA 1998;280(18):1610–5.
[2] Bajaji A. Integrating alternative medicine into practice. JAMA 1998;280(18):1620.
[3] Fontanarosa P. Alternative medicine meets science. JAMA 1998;280(18):1618–9.
[4] Helmes J. Complementary and alternative therapies; a new frontier for nursing education. J Nurs Educ 2006;45(3):117–22.
[5] Cohen M. Complementary and alternative medicine: legal boundaries and regulatory perspectives. Baltimore (MD): John Hopkins Press; 1998.
[6] Hamowy R. The early development of medical licensing laws in the United States: 1875–1900. J Libert Stud 1979;3(1):73.
[7] Rothstein W. American medical schools and the practice of medicine: a history. New York: Oxford University Press; 1987.
[8] Coulter H. Divided legacy: the conflict between homeopathy and the American Medical Association. Berkeley (CA): North Atlantic Books; 1973.
[9] Holder V. From handmaiden to right hand—the infancy of nursing. AORN J 2004;79(2): 376–80.
[10] McDonald L. Florence Nightingale, an introduction to her life and family. Waterloo (Belgium): Wilfred Laurier University Press; 2001.
[11] Nightingale F. Notes on nursing: what it is and what it is not. New York: Dover; 1969.
[12] Hilliard J, Johnson M. State practice acts of licensed health professions: scope of practice. DePaul J Health Care Law 2004;237–56.
[13] Chicago National League Ball Club Inc. v Thompson, 483 N.E.2d 1245, 1250, 1985.
[14] Allgeyer v Louisiana, 165 U.S. 578 (1897).
[15] National Center for Complementary/Alternative Medicine. 2006. Available at: http://www.nccam.nih.gov. Accessed November 13, 2006.

[16] Cohen M. Holistic health care: influencing alternative and complementary medicine in insurance and regulatory schemes. Ariz Law Rev 1996;83–152.

[17] Van Hemel P. A way out of the maze: federal agency preemption of state licensing and regulation of complementary and alternative medicine practitioners. Am J Law Med 2001; 329–44.

[18] Hadley E. Nurses and prescriptive authority: a legal and economic analysis. Am J Law Med 1989;15(2–3):245–99.

[19] Bullough B. The first two phases of nursing licensure. In: Hadley, E, editor. Nurses and prescriptive authority: a legal and economic analysis. Am J Law Med 1984;15:245–99.

[20] Florida Statute §464.001, Part I.

[21] Oregon Statute ORS §678.010.

[22] Texas occupations code and statutes regulating the practice of nursing (2006) Chapter 301.

[23] Sparber A. State boards of nursing and scope of practice of registered nurses: performing complementary therapies. Online J Issues Nurs 2001;6(3). Available at: http://www.nursing world.org/ojin/topic15/tpc15, 2001. Accessed November 14, 2006.

[24] Eskinazi D. Factors that shape alternative medicine. JAMA 1998;280(18):1621–3.

[25] American Medical Association House of Delegates. Resolution 306 (A-06) (2006).

[26] Sussman D. Holistic nursing: NP programs at UCSF first to include alternative therapies in curriculum. Newsweek 2000;13(8):31.

[27] Frisch N. Nursing as a context for alternative/complementary modalities. Online J Issues Nurs 2001;6(2). Available at: http://www.nursingworld.org/ojin/topic15, 2001. Accessed November 13, 2006.

[28] Watson J. Postmodern nursing and beyond. London: Churchill Livingstone; 2000.

[29] George J. Nursing theory: the base for professional practice. 5th edition. Stanford (CT): Appleton & Lange; 2002.

[30] American Association of Colleges of Nursing. The essentials of master's education for advanced practice nursing. Washington, DC: American Association of Colleges of Nursing; 1996.

[31] NANDA. Nursing diagnosis: definitions and classification, 2003–2004. Philadelphia: NANDA; 2004.

[32] McClosky J, Bulichek G. Nursing interventions classification (NIC): Iowa intervention project. 4th edition. St. Louis (MO): Mosby; 2003.

[33] Moorhead S, Johnson M, Maas M. Nursing outcomes classificatio (NOC): Iowa intervention project. 3rd edition. St. Louis (MO): Mosby; 2003.

[34] American Medical Association. Policy H-480. Unconventional medical care in the United States. BOT Rep. 15-A-94.

[35] American Medical Association Resolution 306 (A-06); H-480. Alternative medicine.

[36] American Holistic Nurses Certification Corporation. 2006. Available at: http://ahncc/ natureofannca3.htm. Accessed November 13, 2006.

[37] Executive Order No. 13,147. 65 Federal Register 13, 233 (March 7, 2000).

[38] White House Commission on Complementary and Alternative Medicine. Final report 2002. Available at: http://govinfo.library.unit.edu/whc.camp/pdfs/fr2002. Accessed November 13, 2006.

[39] Boozang K. National policy on CAM: the White House commission report. J Law Med Ethics 2003;31:251–71.

[40] Noah L, Noah B. Health care in America: a new generation of challenges: a drug by any other name? 17 Stanford Law and Policy Review 165 (2006).

[41] Stockwell v Washington State, 622 P.2d 910; Nurville v Mississippi State Medical Association, 364 So.2d 1084.

[42] Peters R. The effectiveness of therapeutic touch: a meta-analytic review. Nurs Sci Q 1999; 12(1):52–61.

[43] Rowland A. Intuitive Reiki for our times: essential techniques for enhancing your practice. Reiki News 2006;5(2):47–50.

[44] Miller R. Problems in health care law. Sudbury (MA): Jones & Bartlett; 2006.

[45] In re: Guess 393 S.E. 2d 833 (1990 North Carolina).

[46] Charrell v Gonzales, 660 NYS2d 665 (1977).

[47] Kapp M. Patient autonomy in the age of consumer-driven health care: informed consent and informed choice. 2 Journal of Health and Biomedical Law 1 (2006).

[48] Vlasis R. The doctor is out, or unconventional methods for healing: resolving the standard of care for an alternative medicine practitioner. 43 Houston Law Review 495 (2006).

[49] Craft v Peebles, 893 P2d 138, 149; Brown v Shyne, 151 N.E. 197, 199 (New York 1926).

[50] Parker v Wolinsky-Friedlan (2003). No. CV020470262 Connecticut Superior Court. December 4, 2003.

[51] Fleisher L, Dechene J. Telemedicine and E-Health law. New York: Law Journal Press; 2006.

ELSEVIER
SAUNDERS

NURSING
CLINICS
OF NORTH AMERICA

Nurs Clin N Am 42 (2007) 213–228

Holistic Assessment and Care: Presence in the Process

Pamela J. Potter, DNSc, ARNP[a],*,
Noreen Frisch, PhD, RN, FAAN, APHN[b]

[a]Biobehavioral Nursing and Health Systems, University of Washington,
Box 357266, Seattle, WA 98195–7266, USA
[b]Cleveland State University, 2121 Euclid Avenue, Cleveland, OH 44115, USA

Holistic assessment and care are inseparable from the nursing process and are effectively described within the context of the holistic caring process (HCP). The HCP is a circular model of nursing practice that allows for reflecting concurrently on every aspect of the nurse-person interaction [1]. The HCP is established through attention to each of nursing's practice domains: cognitive, affective, and experiential. Further, the HCP is guided by holistic philosophy and theory and can be documented in standardized nursing languages.

The HCP is an extension of (or rather an elaboration on) the five-step nursing process known to most nurses. The HCP invites a nurse to enter into the client's world; to use qualitative and quantitative data and reflective techniques to come to understand the client, his needs, and wants; and then to plan care based on a holistic understanding of each individual. The purpose of this article is to place nursing in the context of holistic practice; to explicate the role of presence as an essential condition for holistic care; and to provide an example of the HCP that incorporates theory, presence, and practice documented in the standard formats.

Nursing as holistic practice

Holistic nursing practice informed by a philosophy of holism emphasizes a "sensitive balance between art and science, analytic and intuitive skills, self-care skills, and the ability to care for patients using the

---

* Corresponding author.
E-mail address: potterpj@u.washington.edu (P.J. Potter).

interconnectedness of body, mind and spirit" [2]. Holistic nursing practice includes the nurse as coparticipant within holistic care, necessitating the personal integration of self-care as a requisite for holistic practice. Self-awareness gained allows for recognition of a greater interconnectedness with all beings and, in the nurse-person encounter, becomes a tool for facilitating healing. Holistic nursing practice is relationship centered, a nurse-person collaboration for care.

Such practice draws on knowledge, theories, expertise, intuition, and creativity [3]. These elements of holistic nursing practice can be organized under three domains: cognitive, experiential, and affective (Table 1). Knowledge and theory provide cognitive tools for reflective practice. Expertise, an experiential tool, evolves from actual practice, multiple unique nurse-person encounters within the health care context. The affective tools of intuition and creativity express the art of holistic nursing practice, allowing the nurse to feel, experience, and follow inner guidance within the context of the nurse-person relationship [4].

Knowledge

The HCP is informed by nursing knowledge, beginning with that which is required for licensure. The holistic nurse must have broad knowledge of the discipline, its practices, and its specialties. Nursing knowledge is grounded in the disciplines of the basic and social sciences, informed by professional values and applied in professional practice [4]. The holistic nurse acquires a foundation of knowledge in the biomedical and psychosocial sciences as well as in the liberal arts, including philosophy, art, music, drama, language, religion, ethics, and history.

Nursing knowledge acquired in biomedical education is culturally informed by that context, reflecting what one knows about the physiologic, psychologic, and social (biopsychosocial) functioning of human beings, primarily in terms of biologic outcomes and secondarily in terms of interpersonal relationships and quality of life. Further, giving and evaluating

Table 1
Elements of nursing practice and practice domains

Element	Domain	Use in practice
Knowledge	Cognitive	Understanding the health and disease states; interpreting regimens of care
Theory	Cognitive	Reflection, considered judgments
Expertise	Experiential	Skilled performance
Intuition	Affective	Subjective knowing
Creativity	Affective	Spontaneity; solving problems or challenges

From Frisch NC. Nursing theory in holistic nursing practice. In: Dossey BM, Keegan L, Guzzetta CE, editors. Holistic nursing: a handbook for practice. 4th edition. Boston (MA): Jones and Bartlett Publishers; 2005. p. 81; with permission.

nursing care are formulated in terms of achieving physiologic balance, which, in turn, has an impact on biopsychosocial functioning. Skills necessary to carry out the activities of contemporary nursing are those of observation, measurement, and technical proficiency in basic intervention techniques. Without meeting these rudimentary knowledge standards through education and licensure, a person offering care to another within the realm of contemporary Western health care cannot legally or ethically call herself or himself a "nurse."

Holistic nursing knowledge transcends and includes biomedicine, applying principles of mind-body and spiritual dimensions to understanding of health and healing. This knowledge informs the holistic nurse's understanding of complementary or alternative therapies and practices that a client might use to affect improved health. Such therapies include alternative medical systems like Ayurveda and Oriental medicine, mind-body therapies like progressive-muscle relaxation and guided imagery, and herbal and dietary therapies. This larger knowledge paradigm supports speculation about the spiritual as well as bioaction pathways of energy therapies, such as Reiki, Healing Touch, and Therapeutic Touch.

Theory

Theory is the framework or world view of the nurse. Theory permits the nurse to make sense of observed data because theory helps one to understand events within a coherent framework. Further, use of theory guides the nurse to identify the assumptions used to interpret data and to plan practice interventions [4]. The holistic nurse, drawing on nursing theory or nursing informed theory to guide practice, chooses a theoretic framework most suitable to holistic philosophy. Nursing theory-guided practice integrates theory, research, and practice, creating a container in which the nurse-person encounter takes place. "Theory-guided practice is not simply the means by which nursing theory is applied in the care of patients; it provides a dialogue—between patient and nurse, the empirical and theoretical —by which situation-specific knowledge about health and healing can be generated" [5]. Theory provides the interpretive matrix for clinical judgment for the nurse-person interaction. Application of established nursing theories as practice guides has a positive impact on nursing care. This is demonstrated by increased satisfaction expressed by the care receiver and nurse provider. Practice guided by theory offers something different—a nursing perspective—to health care delivery [6].

Expertise

Expertise is the practice component of nursing gained only from experiences with patients, nurses, families, and coworkers in the "real-world" setting. Initially, the novice nurse draws expertise from knowledge founded in the biomedical sciences and experience acquired under the mentorship of expert nurses [7]. The acute clinical setting is often held as the optimal site for gaining nursing expertise, possibly because it offers examples of break-downs in biophysiologic and psychologic function and opportunity for rapid application of technical skills with immediate evaluative confirmation of the effectiveness of those skills. Yet, nursing practice occurs in a variety of settings, and nursing expertise extends beyond technical competence.

Expertise can be described "as an ability to use multiple forms of know-ing, plus use of self, in a seamless way to promote care that is tailor-made for the patient" [8]. Hardy and colleagues [8] identified four enabling practice expertise factors:

Reflectivity: continually reconsiders, reassesses, and reframes care within a changing context
Practice organization: prioritizes and orders activities to use nurse-person interactions effectively to engage everyone in care
Autonomy and authority: accepts responsibility and demonstrates confidence in decision making
Interpersonal relationships: demonstrates intentional effort to create successful working relationships

The complexity of human beings warrants that "expert nurses, particu-larly those who see themselves as holistic, need to have a breadth of ad-vanced knowledge and skills" [9]. Experience is at the root of expertise. Life experiences, knowledge, and clinical experience all inform each other. In addition to conventional Western medicine, the holistic nurse has knowl-edge and expertise in complementary and alternative modalities. Holistic nursing standards of practice and advanced practice form the basis for certification that recognizes and acknowledges nursing practice expertise incorporating multiple ways of knowing.

Intuition

Intuition is the aspect of practice based on insights that emerge from connections with people and builds on experiences of similar and like cases. Intuition has been described as a process of knowing more than one can explain [10]. Nursing intuition occurs as "integration of forms of knowing in a sudden realization" [11]. Intuition precipitates analytic processes facil-itating caring action. "Intuitive perception allows one to know something immediately without consciously using reason" [12]. Young [13] described intuition as a "process by which we know something about a client which cannot be verbalized or is verbalized poorly or for which the source of the knowledge cannot be determined." Intuition may be a visceral feeling of something wrong requiring action, even though no obvious evidence supports the feeling [14]. Rew [15] categorized nursing intuition as cognitive, gestalt, or precognitive processes. Cognitive inference reaches conclusions from rapidly processing cues. Gestalt intuition apprehends whole pattern. Precognitive intuition, suggesting a possible energy field interaction, perceives change before it happens.

Effken [16] describes nursing intuition as direct perception of environmental information or higher order variables calling for action. Such higher order variables go unnoticed by the novice. This offers some explanation as to how the expert nurse who perceives these variables may not be able to describe underlying lower order properties accurately or how new information outside of the realm of the nurse's experience may be intuitively interpreted and acted on. Through intuition as direct perception, the expert nurse, like a "smart device," is sensitive to and capable of immediately apprehending and acting on higher order information.

The holistic nurse is intuitive, cultivating awareness beyond the five senses. Intuition looks beyond the obvious and comes from a deeper level of knowing that accommodates the barometer of feelings, a processing of information that recognizes the impact of subtle awareness on the greater whole. More than a hunch or a vague uneasy feeling, intuition in nursing is informed by knowledge, theory, and expertise and is cultivated by self-knowledge. Self-knowledge allows the nurse to interpret whether or not an intuitive insight stems from personal concerns or from a higher level of nurse-person communication. Although intuitive judgment increases proportionately with nursing expertise, it may also be observed and cultivated in the novice nurse. Further perceiving that all people may experience intuitive insights, the intuitive nurse attends to and, when appropriate, acts on client/patient perceptions [14].

Creativity

Creativity is the art of nursing—the ability to meet client needs spontaneously. Creativity permits the nurse to individualize care and promote an aesthetic environment. Within creativity, the nurse-person relationship occurs not within knowledge, theory, or expertise, although they provide explanatory value. Creativity is an awakening and cultivation of imagination. Creativity "requires uncovering the heart, opening the mind, letting loose the imagination, creating an environment conducive to creativity, working to master a form, and demonstrating the courage to take risks and be vulnerable" [17]. Holistic nurses practicing the art of nursing draw from their innermost selves to master the physical "form" of nursing, which manifests in "acts of caring."

Gaydos [17] describes the art of nursing as a cocreative aesthetic process with four aspects: engagement, mutuality, movement, and new form. Engagement is the initiation of a relationship, wherein participants value the process and each other. Mutuality, the interpenetration of experience, one with another, is observable in relational qualities demonstrating trust, warmth, confidence, credibility, honesty, expectation, courtesy, and respect.

Movement is within and through. Movement within is characterized by rhythm, a syncopated moving between self and other. Movement through is demonstrated as a temporal pattern moving recursively through beginning to middle to end, from the unknown to the known, and from unformed to form. New forms—physical, psychosocial, linguistic, intellectual, or transpersonal—are cocreated out of the dynamic mutual nurse-person relationship.

Creativity vitalizes holistic practice, enhancing therapeutic value and capacity for healing in all participants. Through creativity, the art of nursing can be observed and appreciated. Such encounters produce a healing environment for the client and professional pride and satisfaction for the nurse.

Nursing as presence

Presence is essential to the healing relationship. Presence is the application of the art of nursing. Presence is the ability of the nurse to recognize that the nurse-person encounter is a mutual dynamic with two people bringing all that they are, recognized and unrecognized, to the encounter. More than just showing up, presence is the capability to empathize, listen, reflect, and observe—to be with the client in the moment and not somewhere else. Dossey and Guzzetta [18] describe presence as a way of doing the following:

Approaching an individual that respects and honors her or his essence
Relating that reflects a quality of being with and in collaboration with rather than doing to
Entering into a shared experience (or field of consciousness) that promotes healing potentials and an experience of well-being

Presence is "a multidimensional state of being available in a situation with the wholeness of one's individual being. It is a holistic self-giving exchange, the acknowledgment of a sacred quality operating within one person that can intentionally connect with that sacred quality in others" [19]. McKivergin [19] describes three levels of holistic nursing presence, including physical, psychologic, and therapeutic. The essence of physical presence is "being there" in the action of physical service and involves routine nursing as well as complex interventions performed at the level of the physical. Presence at this level requires fundamental nursing knowledge and technical clinical expertise. The challenge for the holistic nurse at this level is to bracket personal life concerns and give intentional focus to caring for the client physically. Psychologic presence, "being with" the person, requires a higher level of presence—therapeutic use of self to offer comfort and support while drawing on psychosocial and self-knowledge/expertise to provide an opportunity for the client to interpret and find meaning within a particular life event. Therapeutic presence is holistic presence—using the total resources of body, mind, emotions, and spirit—wherein the nurse-person relationship is one of relating as whole being to whole being. This level of presence transcends and includes the first two levels, fully inviting the affective elements of intuition and creativity.

Through presence, the holistic nurse, reflecting possibilities for health and well-being, acts as a mirror in which the person may look as he or she seeks to discover ways to find his or her own health and well-being. The reflection can only be as clear as the mirror. All healing happens within the person. Through presence, the holistic nurse creates the environment for facilitating the discovery of healing within the self.

Nursing as holistic caring process

The nursing process was originally described as the "work" of nursing, a linear process of steps used to fulfill the purposes of nursing [1]. The HCP, an adaptation and expansion of the nursing process, incorporates the standards of holistic nursing practice into a circular model of process with the nurse-person interaction at its core (Fig. 1). This process incorporates several phases that may occur simultaneously: assessment, pattern/problems/needs, outcomes, therapeutic care plan, implementation, and evaluation. The phases act as organizing principles, providing a fluid structure for planning and documenting nursing care and the client's response to

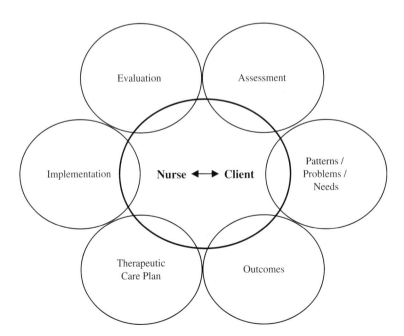

Fig. 1. Circular model of the HCP.

that care [14]. Identified patterns provide the structure for creating mutual goals and evaluating responses to actions initiated within the process.

The application of holistic nursing philosophy to nursing adds a whole person perspective to the process. The process is relational, wherein the whole person—biopsychosocial-spiritual—is recognized as a mutual participant in the nurse-person interaction. Within the person-centered process, insight into the lived experience of health and well-being is gained through eliciting the person's perceptions of reality and life's meaning. Natural and human sciences, qualitative and quantitative data, inform the process. A nursing theoretic framework compatible with holism completes the HCP. Data are gathered, and care is evaluated and documented in the language of theory. The HCP provides a systematic process for practicing holistic nursing, a structure to guide the novice and the experienced nurse [14].

Documentation of nursing care requires a professional vocabulary for justifying and describing caregiving activities and outcomes and meets the legal requirement for keeping records of care provided [14]. Nurse educators and practitioners, endeavoring to establish nursing as a distinct health care profession with billable services, have established standardized nursing languages. The taxonomies of nursing practice developed in North America link nursing diagnosis, nursing interventions, and nursing outcomes classifications into a comprehensive list compatible with computerized documentation and inclusion in standardized multidisciplinary vocabularies [20]. These taxonomies provide an atheoretic standardized language structure that is compatible with a holistic perspective [21]. The holistic nurse may use these standardized languages creatively to document the breadth and depth of care given.

Holistic assessment

> Holistic nurses assess each person holistically using appropriate conventional and holistic methods while the uniqueness of the person is honored [22].

During assessment, the information-gathering phase, the nurse collaborates with the client to appraise the overall pattern of responses to identify health patterns and prioritize concerns [14]. Family, other health care professionals, and diagnostic data provide supplemental information. The assessment phase is a cultural exchange of expert knowledge, wherein the nurse and client bring expertise to the exchange [23]. Within this process, the nurse acknowledges the influence of his or her own patterns on the healing relationship. The person assessed is considered to be the primary information source and interpreter of meaning. Through interpersonal interaction, observation, and measurement, the nurse gleans information about the client's patterns. Interpersonal interaction reveals health patterns as identified by the client. Information perceived by the physical senses (possibly including energy field assessment) plus intuition comprise nursing observation. Measurement, quantifiable information obtained from instruments, provides evidence to corroborate or refute observation. Holistic assessment, an ongoing process, provides continuous data for identifying pattern changes that occur over time. Assessment data are documented in the client's record. New information provided during each nurse-person encounter helps to explain relationships, may validate previously collected data and conclusions, and serves to guide the caring process.

Pattern identification

> Holistic nurses identify and prioritize each person's actual and potential patterns/challenges/needs and life processes related to health, wellness, disease, or illness, which may or may not facilitate well being [22].

Within the HCP, the nurse uses standardized language to describe a person's patterns[14].This language must be understandable to those involved in the person's care: nurses, other health care professionals, the managed care provider, and the person receiving nursing care. Nursing diagnosis within the North American Nursing Diagnosis Association (NANDA) taxonomy provides standardized language for describing pattern and is defined as "a clinical judgment about the individual, family, or community responses to actual and potential health problems/life processes" [24]. The diagnostic statement consists of two parts: the diagnostic label plus related factors. The diagnostic label describes an identifiable pattern from one of 13 functional domains, as listed in Box 1. Multiaxial in structure, every diagnostic statement explicitly or implicitly incorporates each of seven axes listed

---

Box 1. Domains of nursing diagnosis

Domain 1: health promotion
Domain 2: nutrition
Domain 3: elimination
Domain 4: activity/rest
Domain 5: perception/cognition
Domain 6: self-perception
Domain 7: role relationships
Domain 8: sexuality
Domain 9: coping/stress tolerance
Domain 10: life principles
Domain 11: safety/protection
Domain 12: comfort
Domain 13: growth/development

Data from North American Nursing Diagnosis Association. Nursing diagnoses: definitions and classification 2005–2006. Philadelphia: NANDA; 2005.

Box 2. Nursing diagnosis taxonomy structure

Axis 1: diagnostic concept
Axis 2: time (acute, chronic, intermittent, continuous)
Axis 3: unit of care (individual, family, group, community)
Axis 4: age (fetus to old-old adult)
Axis 5: health status (wellness, risk, actual)
Axis 6: descriptor (limits or specifies the meaning of the
    diagnostic concept)
Axis 7: topology (parts/regions of the body)

Data from North American Nursing Diagnosis Association. Nursing diagnoses:
definitions and classification 2005–2006. Philadelphia: NANDA; 2005.

in Box 2. Of particular relevance to holistic assessment, the health status axis reflects the position or rank on a health continuum from wellness to illness, accommodating actual, risk, and wellness diagnoses. "Actual" conveys present time, "risk" suggests vulnerability, and "wellness" reflects a quality of health resulting from deliberate effort and suggests the possibility for enhancement. The trifocal model (Fig. 2) for nursing diagnosis developed by Kelley and colleagues [25], adapted to include the 13 domains [14], organizes the identified patterns of nursing diagnosis into a comprehensive map. The base of the pyramid represents actual health problems or challenges. The next level, reflecting a higher level of wellness, identifies the client's risk for developing problems. The apex, the highest level of wellness, represents those patterns with potential for enhancement and allows for the possibility of facilitating harmony and balance. As Frisch and Frisch [1] observed, this structure "gives the nurse a framework to use the diagnostic language in all aspects of nursing care." This model, accommodating the multidimensionality of the person, allows the nurse to identify and map strengths that may be enhanced in the midst of potential and manifest illness. The diagram provides a motivational tool facilitating a mutual care-planning process.

From the list of diagnoses and defining characteristics, the nurse compares specific diagnostic characteristics with observable cues and inferences gleaned from the assessment process to determine one or more diagnoses fitting the client's pattern [24]. Nurses must draw on all the elements of holistic practice to conclude whether or not the observations sufficiently confirm the existence of a particular health pattern [14]. NANDA nursing diagnoses reflect commonly observed patterns. If not, formulation of a new diagnosis may be required.

Further, standardized language, although meeting cultural requirements for documenting nursing care based on predictable outcomes, does not

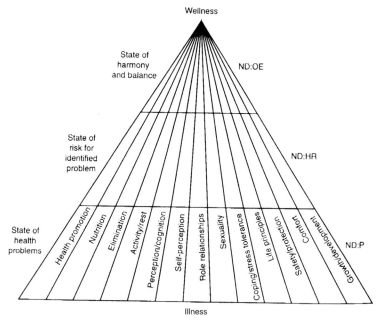

Fig. 2. The trifocal model. HR, high risk; ND, nursing diagnosis; OE, opportunity for enhancement; P, problem. (*Adapted from* Kelley J, Frisch N, Avant K. A trifocal model of nursing diagnosis: wellness revisited. Nurs Diagn 1995;6:125; with permission.)

preclude use of a nursing theoretic framework. Additionally, such documentation favors the possibility of evaluating theory-based practice outcomes. Theory-oriented strategies suggested by Frisch and Kelley [21] include "the use of theory-specific language in the 'related-to' clause of the diagnosis, writing narrative notes along with the standard classifications, and documenting impact of nursing activities on client conditions."

The diagnostic process, whenever possible, is a collaborative one, wherein the nurse validates and prioritizes diagnoses with the recipient of care. The holistic nurse remembers that these descriptions are not the pattern; they are only touchstones for choosing actions that may alter a person's health patterns in the direction of health and well-being.

Outcomes

Holistic nurses specify appropriate outcomes for each person's actual or potential patterns/challenges/needs [22].

As with all the steps of the HCP, the establishment of outcomes is a relational process. "An outcome is a direct statement of a nurse-person identified goal to be achieved within a specific time frame" [14]. Considering objective circumstances and the client's perceptions, chosen outcomes reflect the maximum level of wellness reasonably attainable for the person. Outcomes are measured using standard/known identifiers and characteristics, some of which are objective and some of which are subjective. The taxonomy of outcomes delineated by the Nursing Outcomes Classification (NOC) provides a comprehensive list of observable or measurable outcomes responsive to nursing interventions [26]. These observations can act as indicators of individual change as well as aggregate change for larger population comparisons. Within the taxonomy, NOC outcomes may fit in one of the following categories [14]:

  Circumstances that should or should not occur in the client's status
  Level at which some change should occur
  Client's verbalizations about what he or she knows, understands, or feels
    about the situation
  Specific client behaviors or signs/symptoms that are expected to occur as
    a result of the intervention
  Specific client behaviors that are expected to occur as a result of adequate
    management of the environment

Outcome criteria delineate specific observations or personal statements that indicate outcome achievement. Specified outcomes reflect the nurse-person intervention goals and direct the therapeutic care plan. Nursing interventions with observable milestones for achieving desired changes are chosen in collaboration with the client. Both parties commit to facilitating movement toward those desired changes. In keeping with the theme of the HCP, outcomes are achieved within the collaborative nurse-person relationship. Arbitrary outcomes assigned by the nurse impede outcome achievement. Similarly, rigid adherence to outcomes by either party in the nurse-person relationship fails to recognize the journey with its myriad possibilities for healing.

Therapeutic care plan

  Holistic nurses engage each person to mutually create an appropriate plan
  of care that focuses on health promotion, recovery, restoration, or peaceful
  dying so that the person is as independent as possible [22].

During the planning phase, the holistic nurse assists the client to identify ways for repatterning health behaviors toward well-being. The plan outlines nursing interventions chosen to facilitate achievement of identified outcomes. A nursing intervention is "any direct care treatment that a nurse performs on behalf of a client. The treatments include nurse-initiated treatments resulting from nursing diagnoses, physician-initiated treatments resulting from medical diagnoses, and performance of the daily essential functions for the client who cannot do these" [27]. The Nursing

Interventions Classification (NIC) provides a comprehensive list that includes independent and collaborative direct care interventions performed by nurses in giving patient care [28]. The holistic nurse chooses interventions, validated by efficacy research and feasible to implement, that facilitate achieving desired outcomes, address identified health patterns (nursing diagnoses), and are within the nurse's scope of competency necessary for successful implementation [14].

Holistic nurses incorporate complementary modalities into their practice. To complement standard nursing care, holistic nurses may select complementary therapies and noninvasive nursing interventions [29]. "When a complementary/alternative modality is used to address a concern identified as a nursing diagnosis, the action becomes an identified nursing intervention planned to address/remedy a nursing problem or concern" [30]. These modalities "treat the body (biofeedback, therapeutic massage), relieve the mind (humor, imagery, meditation), comfort the soul (prayer), and support significant interpersonal interaction (healing presence)" [31].

Implementation

> Holistic nurses prioritize each person's plan of holistic care and holistic nursing interventions are implemented accordingly [22].

During the implementation phase, the nurse and client carry out the plan of care. Important factors for implementation include the "awareness that (1) people are active participants in their care; (2) nursing care must be performed with purposeful, focused intention; and (3) a person's humanness is an important factor in implementation" [14]. Krieger [32] wrote that therapeutic use of self offers the greatest potential for facilitating healing. Within the holistic framework, action on any aspect of the biopsychosocial-spiritual being creates a corresponding response in the other aspects. Human emotions are linked to physiologic responses [33]. The act of compassionate touch in the midst of procedural touch yields a psychophysiologic response in the nurse-person encounter changing the consciousness and physiology of both participants.

Evaluation

> Holistic nurses evaluate each person's responses to holistic care regularly and systematically and the continuing holistic nature of the healing process is recognized and honored [22].

Evaluation is a mutual process between the nurse and the recipient of care, a planned review of the nurse-person interaction to identify factors facilitating or hindering anticipated outcomes. Evaluation provides an opportunity to review the biopsychosocial-spiritual data that have been collected and recorded throughout the HCP. Evaluation uses qualitative and quantitative data to compare identified patterns (nursing diagnoses) with outcome criteria to evaluate nursing intervention results. The entire health care team, including the patient as a key participant, evaluates the effectiveness of holistic care. Rather than an evaluation of success or failure, the process offers the nurse and client an opportunity to gain insight into the interconnection of patterns contributing positively or negatively to health and well-being and to identify new possibilities for repatterning behaviors. Evaluation is continuous and contributes to care plan revision with the development of new outcomes. Some outcomes may not be immediately observable or measurable. Evaluation, extending beyond the nurse-person encounter, includes self-aware reflection on the entire HCP by the nurse. From an ecologic perspective, the holistic nurse's reflection includes identifying impact on the health care delivery system, physical environment, and greater society, with implications for professional practice standards and health and environmental policy [14].

Implications of the process

The HCP provides a context and a structure for the nurse-person encounter. Within that encounter, the client draws what is needed or is perceived to be needed. Ultimately, it is the person who heals; actually, each person in the encounter is potentially changed by that encounter in the direction of well-being. By definition, holistic nursing can be practiced in any setting by any nurse. The standards of holistic nursing practice, as organized by the HCP, incorporate easily into subspecialty care standards (eg, critical care and psychiatric subspecialties), ensuring not only quality physical care but quality holistic nursing care for these populations [14]. The nursing process is changed through the lens of the standards of holistic nursing practice. The HCP creates a framework in which to refine and enhance as well as a means to describe and document holistic nursing care. "Holistic nursing is both the practice of presence and the implementation of process" [14]. A holistic approach to nursing integrates process and presence in the provision of care. Process alone is empty without presence. Presence alone is insufficient without the process.

Challenge of holistic practice

"Holistic practice ... is as unique as the individual practicing" [34]. Clinical practice is only one facet of holistic practice. Holistic nursing practice includes health policy, nursing research, philosophic writing, and teaching nursing students. Nursing diagnosis, NIC, and NOC are only words, convenient labels for describing what nursing does, but there are no convenient labels for the actual human interaction between nurse and patient. Holistic theory-guided nursing practice attempts to articulate this interaction. "Unfortunately, curricula in nursing programs worldwide and content in professional nurse registration and certification examinations are still embedded in the medical model, and only a few nurse administrators in health care settings recognize the importance of nursing theory-guided practice as an incentive for recruitment and retention of qualified nurses" [6]. The HCP addresses the need for theory and holism and the need for documentation of what a nurse does. The HCP is performed within the contemporary arena of health care. The goal of the nurse is to facilitate well-being, which comes in many forms ranging from establishing electrolyte balance to supporting peace and joy.

References

[1] Frisch NC, Frisch LE. Psychiatric mental health nursing. 3rd edition. Albany (NY): Delmar; 2005.

[2] Dossey BM, editor. Core curriculum for holistic nursing. Gaithersburg (MD): Aspen Publishers; 1997.

[3] American Holistic Nurses' Association. Description of holistic nursing. Flagstaff (AZ): AHNA; 1998.

[4] Frisch NC. Nursing theory in holistic nursing practice. In: Dossey BM, Keegan L, Guzzetta CE, editors. Holistic nursing: a handbook for practice. 4th edition. Boston: Jones and Bartlett Publishers; 2005. p. 79–90.

[5] Reed PG. The dialogue within nursing theory-guided practice: a frontier of knowledge and development. Nurs Sci Q 2006;19(4):328–9.

[6] Parse RR. Research findings evince benefits of nursing theory-guided practice. Nurs Sci Q 2006;19(2):87.

[7] Benner P. Novice to expert: excellence and power in clinical nursing practice. Reading (MA): Addison-Wesley; 1985.

[8] Hardy S, Titchen A, Manley K, et al. Re-defining nursing expertise in the United Kingdom. Nurs Sci Q 2006;19(3):260–4.

[9] Baumann SL. What does expert nursing practice mean? Nurs Sci Q Jul 2006;19(3):259–60.

[10] Polanyi M. Personal knowledge. New York: Harper & Row; 1958.

[11] King L, Appleton JV. Intuition: a critical review of the research and rhetoric. J Adv Nurs 1997;26(1):194–202.

[12] Schraeder BD, Fischer DK. Using intuitive knowledge in the neonatal intensive care nursery. Holist Nurs Pract 1987;1(3):45–51.

[13] Young CE. Intuition and nursing process. Holist Nurs Pract 1987;1(3):52–62.

[14] Potter PJ, Guzzetta CE. The holistic caring process. In: Dossey BM, Keegan L, Guzzetta CE, editors. Holistic nursing: a handbook for practice. 4th edition. Boston: Jones and Bartlett Publishers; 2005. p. 341–75.

[15] Rew L. Intuition in decision-making. Image J Nurs Sch 1988;20(3):150–4.

[16] Effken JA. Informational basis for expert intuition. J Adv Nurs 2001;34(2):246–55.

[17] Gaydos HLB. The art of holistic nursing and the human health experience. In: Dossey BM, Keegan L, Guzzetta CE, editors. Holistic nursing: a handbook for practice. 4th edition. Boston: Jones and Bartlett Publishers; 2005. p. 57–76.

[18] Dossey BM, Guzzetta CE. Holistic nursing practice. In: Dossey BM, Keegan L, Guzzetta CE, editors. Holistic nursing: a handbook for practice. 4th edition. Boston: Jones and Bartlett Publishers; 2005. p. 5–37.

[19] McKivergin M. The nurse as an instrument of healing. In: Dossey BM, Keegan L, Guzzetta CE, editors. Holistic nursing: a handbook for practice. 4th edition. Boston: Jones and Bartlett Publishers; 2005. p. 233–54.

[20] Johnson M, Bulechek GM, Dochterman JM, et al. NANDA, NOC, and NIC linkages. 2nd edition. Philadelphia: Elsevier-Health Sciences Division; 2005.

[21] Frisch NC, Kelley JH. Nursing diagnosis and nursing theory: exploration of factors inhibiting and supporting simultaneous use. Nurs Diagn 2002;13(2):53–61.

[22] American Holistic Nurses' Association. Standards of holistic nursing practice. Flagstaff (AZ): AHNA; 2003.

[23] Engebretson J, Littleton LY. Cultural negotiation: a constructivist-based model for nursing practice. Nurs Outlook 2001;49(5):223–30.

[24] North American Nursing Diagnosis Association. Nursing diagnoses: definitions and classification 2005–2006. Philadelphia: NANDA; 2005.

[25] Kelley J, Frisch N, Avant K. A trifocal model of nursing diagnosis: wellness reinforced. Nurs Diagn 1995;6(3):123–8.

[26] Moorhead S, Johnson M, Maas ML. Nursing outcomes classification (NOC). 3rd edition. St. Louis: Mosby; 2004.

[27] McCloskey JC, Bulechek GM. Classification of nursing interventions: implications for nursing diagnoses. In: Carroll-Johnson RM, Paquette M, editors. Classification of nursing diagnoses: proceedings of the tenth conference. Philadelphia: Lippincott; 1994. p. 113–25.

[28] Dochterman JM, Bulechek GM. Nursing interventions classification (NIC). 4th edition. Philadelphia: Elsevier-Health Sciences Division; 2003.

[29] Snyder M, Lindquist R, editors. Complementary/alternative therapies in nursing. 4th edition. New York: Springer; 2002.

[30] Frisch NC. Nursing as a context for complementary/alternative modalities. Online J Issues Nurs 2001;6 Manuscript 2. Available at: http://www.nursingworld.org/ojin/topic15/tpc15_2.htm.

[31] Frisch NC. Standards for holistic nursing practice: a way to think about our care that includes complementary and alternative modalities. Online J Issues Nurs 2001;6 Manuscript 4. Available at: http://www.nursingworld.org/ojin/topic15/tpc15_4.htm.

[32] Krieger D. Foundation of holistic health nursing practice. Philadelphia: Lippincott; 1981.

[33] Pert CB. Molecules of emotion: the science behind mind-body medicine. New York: Simon & Schuster; 1999.

[34] Slater V. Holistic nursing practice. J Holist Nurs 2005;23(3):261–3.

ELSEVIER
SAUNDERS

NURSING
CLINICS
OF NORTH AMERICA

Nurs Clin N Am 42 (2007) 229–241

Promoting Behavior Change: Making Healthy Choices in Wellness and Healing Choices in Illness—Use of Self-Determination Theory in Nursing Practice

Vicki D. Johnson, MSN, RN, CNAA

College of Education and Human Services, School of Nursing, Cleveland State University,
2121 Euclid Avenue, RT 915, Cleveland, OH 44115, USA

It is self-evident that teaching is integral to nursing practice and that nurses often struggle with issues of teaching efficacy as they attempt to educate clients about the importance of adopting healthier behaviors [1–4]. Nurses understand that unhealthy behavior choices, such as poor nutrition, sedentary lifestyle, substance misuse, ineffective stress management, and nonadherence to therapeutic regimens, cause and exacerbate chronic illnesses, and nurses are dedicated to teaching this information to their clients. Nevertheless, it seems that no matter how hard nurses work at teaching clients about healthy lifestyle change, many clients seem unable or unwilling to adopt and maintain these health practices [5]. This problem has significant implications. Bandura [6] states: "We are pouring massive resources into medicalising the ravages of detrimental health habits." Although this problem may be framed in terms of economic and policy issues, it may also be viewed in a humanistic way by examining the toll of just one category of chronic illness on human life—cardiovascular disease.

Cardiovascular disease is the number one cause of death in men and women in the United States. According to the American Heart Association, almost 2500 Americans die of cardiovascular disease each day and cardiovascular disease kills more people than the next four leading causes of death combined [7]. These statistics are all the more sobering when one considers that many of the risk factors for cardiovascular disease are preventable. In fact, experts agree that the best approach to reducing cardiovascular

E-mail address: v.d.johnson01@csuohio.edu

0029-6465/07/$ - see front matter © 2007 Published by Elsevier Inc.
doi:10.1016/j.cnur.2007.02.003   *nursing.theclinics.com*

morbidity and mortality is "full participation from the patient who must adopt and adhere to therapeutic modalities—whether life habit changes or drug therapy" [8]. Furthermore, there is consensus that primary prevention should begin with children as well as adults [9]. Primary prevention includes the identification and elimination of modifiable cardiovascular risk factors—in other words, the adoption and maintenance of healthy lifelong behaviors. Despite easily accessible knowledge about modifiable risk factors, only 3% of women in the Nurses Health Study were engaged in the healthy behaviors of maintaining a desirable body weight, eating a healthy diet, exercising regularly, not smoking, and moderating alcohol intake. Authors of this same study estimate that these healthy behaviors could account for an 84% reduction in heart disease [10,11]. Based on this information, it is clear that knowledge of risk factors alone is not sufficient to motivate behavior change.

Some authors suggested that patient compliance with medical regimens and adoption of healthy behaviors increased when multidisciplinary teams and behavioral interventions were used in several multisite clinical trials. These trials include the Multiple Risk Factor Intervention Trial Research Group (MRFIT), Hypertension Detection and Follow-up Program Cooperative Group (HDFP), and Systolic Hypertension in the Elderly Program (SHEP) [12–14]. These same results have not been demonstrated in clinical practice, however [5]. The reason for this discrepancy is that teaching patients about risk modification, although certainly desirable, is not sufficient to motivate people to change their behaviors. Nurses and other health care providers must also learn to use appropriate strategies to motivate their clients to learn, adopt, and maintain lifelong healthy behaviors.

Therefore, the purpose of this article is to describe alternative and more efficacious strategies for holistic nurses to promote long-term healthy behavior choices in their clients. These strategies are derived from empirical research studies in the fields of psychology, education, and medicine that fall within the context of self-determination theory (SDT). The following section of this article provides a brief overview of SDT [15–17]. This is followed by a concise review of important findings from the research literature that support the usefulness of this strategy in motivating people to adopt and maintain long-term healthy behavior changes and a summary of strategies that holistic nurses can use in varied practice settings (Table 1).

Self-determination theory

> This above all: to thine own self be true
>
> And it must follow, as the night the day
>
> Thou cans't not be false to any man [18].

SDT is a motivational theory based on the organismic perspective that people have an inherent inclination to act on their world, to participate in

Table 1
Examples of nursing interventions to motivate behavior change

Nursing interventions	Example(s)
Use client-centered autonomy-supportive behaviors that provide a rationale for the behavior change	"Following a low-fat diet decreases your risk of heart disease."
Acknowledge that the client might be feeling ambivalent	"You may be feeling that you do not want to follow a low-fat diet."
Use low-pressure language and style	"It's your choice. You are free to decide whether you want to change your diet or not and to what extent."
Remember that the client is responsible for behavior change; the nurse's responsibility is to be present, to be patient, and to support the client in making an informed choice	"I'm more than willing to talk with you about this further. Here are my telephone number and office hours." "How can I best support you in making a decision?"
Avoid coercion, persuasion, punishments, and controlling; give rewards in a noncontrolling manner (eg, as an acknowledgment of good performance) Use wise feedback	"I notice that you kept an accurate record of your dietary intake for the past month, and it shows that you have decreased your fat consumption to 25% of your daily calories. You have also decreased your intake of saturated fats to lower than the level recommended by the US Department of Agriculture. I am confident that you will be able to maintain this reduction for the long term, and you will likely see an improvement in your blood lipid test result. Nice job!"
Establish a therapeutic relationship that supports the client's need for relatedness	"I want to take time to listen to your thoughts and feelings about beginning an exercise program."
Attempt to elicit change talk	"Do you want to quit smoking?" "Have you attempted to stop smoking before? What was that like?" "Does this change seem attainable to you?"
Offer information the client may not be aware of; do not coerce with threatening information	"There are several medications available that are helpful for people who are addicted to nicotine." "Here is where you can learn more about this subject if you would care to."
Support the client's autonomy by facilitating free choice among alternatives	"Which of these options, if any, seem possible for you?" "Do any of these options seem attractive to you?"

activities that interest them, and to integrate these activities into "an ever expanding and more unified representation of who they are" [15]. The theory posits that internalization of motivations (or self-regulation) is an active activity and that this process occurs in harmony with the satisfaction of three innate needs for autonomy, competence, and relatedness. Satisfaction of these psychologic needs is necessary for successful integration (development), self-regulation (self-motivation), and psychologic and physical health and well-being [15–17].

Inherent needs

Autonomy

Autonomy, also known as self-determination, is a fundamental construct in SDT. Autonomy is an inherent psychologic need to act freely according to one's inner self [15]. Another way of thinking about autonomy is to remember the Shakespearean adage: "This above all: to thine own self be true" [18]. An individual possesses "a natural tendency toward authenticity" and is more inclined to behave in a way that is congruent with his or her innermost self [15,17].

It is important to understand that any situation undermining a person's autonomy and causing one to feel controlled decreases intrinsic motivation. Therefore, autonomy support, or bolstering individual autonomy, is crucial to self-motivation and self-regulation. Autonomy support involves understanding the other person's perspective as well as encouraging self-knowledge and the natural processes of self-initiated activity and discovery. Autonomy support is not the same as "permissiveness." In fact, autonomy support may include setting limits but in a way that does not undermine or control the individual. One can "encourage responsibility without undermining authenticity" [15].

Competence

Within SDT, competence is another inherent psychologic need that supports intrinsically motivated behavior and extrinsically motivated behavior. "Feeling competent at a task is an important aspect of one's intrinsic satisfaction. The feeling of being effective is satisfying in its own right, and can even represent the primary draw for a lifelong career" [15]. Satisfaction of the need for competence provides a catalyst for action, and it works hand-in-hand with autonomy to foster self-motivation [15]. In fact, feeling competent does not promote self-motivation unless it is accompanied by feelings of autonomy [17]. Competence is closely related to the concept of self-efficacy—a person believing that he or she has the means to control his or her own behaviors. Some research consistent with social-cognitive theory suggests that self-efficacy is a useful predictor for self-regulatory skills, such as risk factor reduction [6,19].

There is no published research comparing the construct validity of self-efficacy and competence. One correlational study did analyze the constructs of autonomy and self-efficacy in relation to dietary management and satisfaction among people with diabetes. This research found that autonomy was significantly more associated with life satisfaction, whereas self-efficacy was significantly more associated with adherence. This suggests that the constructs of autonomy and self-efficacy are complementary rather than competitive [20].

The National Institutes of Health Behavior Change Consortium (BCC) is a national initiative investigating behavior change theories. One aspect of its mission is to compare and contrast behavior change theories for the purpose of advancing our knowledge about why people adopt certain health behaviors and how health care personnel can best motivate these processes [21,22]. Sponsoring agencies provided $8 million annually from 1999 through 2002 to fund 15 research grants. Three of the 15 research proposals were grounded in SDT. A link to the summary report of the BCC's research projects and findings can be found at the National Institutes of Health Web site [23,24]. The three studies aimed at testing the efficacy of SDT in practice all reported success in eliciting behavior change over a 6- to 18-month time frame. Specifically, one study found that automated telephone counseling worked as well as human counseling by telephone to elicit and sustain a statistically significant increase in activity levels for 6 months. Another study, "Partners for Life," provides evidence that a couples' intervention improves and sustains adherence to dietary, medication, and exercise programs. Couples also demonstrated significant improvement in depressive symptoms and relationship satisfaction, suggesting that partners and clients are pleased with the changes they made. The third study highlights the importance of provider autonomy support and client levels of autonomy and competence in sustaining tobacco cessation at 6, 12, and 18 months. Overall recommendations from the summary report call for further collaborative initiatives to find common ground across behavior change theories and practices. Designated subgroups in the consortium are working in the areas of common conceptual mediators, methodology and data analysis, motivational interviewing, nutrition, physical activity, recruitment and retention, representativeness and translation, tobacco cessation, transbehavioral outcomes assessment, and treatment fidelity [23].

Relatedness

Relatedness refers to "the need to love and be loved, to care and be cared for" [15]. The inherent need for relatedness has not been studied as extensively as the needs for autonomy and competence, particularly among patient populations. There is evidence that intrinsic motivation thrives in environments that provide secure and supportive relationships, however [15,17]. For example, in one study, increased levels of autonomy and relatedness support predicted greater well-being among nursing home residents [17]. In another study, increases in employee performance and well-being at work were predicted by satisfaction of the psychologic needs for autonomy, competence, and relatedness [17]. In contrast, levels of intrinsic motivation in students are lower in settings in which students perceive their teachers as uncaring and uninvolved [15,17,25].

Admittedly, intrinsic motivation may also exist outside of relational contexts, because people are often motivated to engage in interesting projects independently of others. Therefore, relatedness is not considered essential for intrinsic motivation, but it does lend support to intrinsic motivation [17]. Within SDT, however, relatedness is considered important for extrinsic motivations:

> Because extrinsically motivated behaviors are not typically interesting, the primary reason people initially perform such actions is because the behaviors are prompted, modeled, or valued by significant others to whom they feel (or want to feel) attached or related. This suggests that relatedness, the need to feel belongingness and connectedness with others, is centrally important for internalization [17].

The importance of relatedness in motivating extrinsic self-regulation has significant implications for nurses and other health care providers in their interactions with clients in health care settings. Providers who engage in genuine caring behaviors and take time to listen to their clients and to understand the client's experience are more successful in meeting the client's needs for relatedness, autonomy, and competence. Therefore, the client is more successful in internalizing the importance and value of the provider's message and, in turn, is more likely to adopt and sustain the behavior [16,17,26].

Types of self-motivation/self-regulation

SDT is unique in its differentiation of several types of self-motivation. It postulates a continuum of motivations, with "amotivation" on the far left and "intrinsic motivation" on the far right. Four types of "extrinsic motivation" (external regulation, introjected regulation, identified regulation, and integrated regulation) are found between these two poles, with integrated regulation being closest to intrinsic motivation (Fig. 1). Intrinsic motivation is concerned with doing an activity because it is interesting or enjoyable and it provides satisfaction of the basic needs. This means that "the extent to which a person engages in an activity is the function of the extent to which they experience need satisfaction while engaged in the activity" [15–17].

Research findings on the factors that foster or hinder intrinsic motivation run counter to commonly held assumptions and contradict other psychologic research [15,17,27]. For example, research shows that intrinsic motivation is reduced by the use of extrinsic rewards that are perceived as controlling, and therefore detrimental to a person's autonomy. Results of a thorough meta-analysis demonstrate that deadlines, imposed goals, surveillance, threats, orders, and pressured evaluations all undermine intrinsic

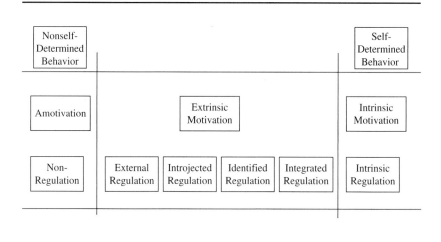

Fig. 1. Types of behavior, motivation, and regulation in SDT. (*Adapted from* Ryan RM, Deci EL. Self-determination theory and the facilitation of intrinsic motivation, social development, and well-being. Am Psychol 2000;55:72; with permission.)

motivation [15,17]. It is also important for the nurse to use noncontrolling language when giving feedback. If feedback messages are construed as controlling, thus diminishing autonomy, intrinsic motivation suffers. Choice is another key factor in autonomy support, and even small opportunities for choice can enhance intrinsic motivation [15].

It is highly probable that healthy behaviors are extrinsically motivated and, to varying degrees, that they are intrinsically motivated. For example, eating a low-calorie diet is not interesting and enjoyable in its own right. If a person wants to lose weight to improve his or her health and recognizes that the low-calorie diet helps in losing weight, however, in SDT terms, he or she has "internalized its regulation" and "more fully accepted it" as his or her own. This person is more likely to stay on the low-calorie diet than an individual who is not interested in dieting but was told by a doctor that he or she must follow a diet [16]. The process of internalization is enhanced by satisfaction of the basic needs for autonomy, competence, and relatedness. This is an important concept, and it has significant implications for motivating people to adopt and maintain healthy behaviors or to practice self-management of medical regimens [26].

A complete explication of SDT is beyond the scope of this article, as is a thorough review of the 30 years of research literature that supports its theoretic constructs. Such a thorough review is not necessary to understand the importance of SDT in motivating people to engage in and maintain healthy behaviors, however. The next section of this article provides a partial review of the research literature and proposes a succinct strategy based on empirical evidence to promote long-term healthy behaviors.

Empirical support for the efficacy of self-determination theory in health care

Research demonstrates that the predominant method of decision making in health care is paternalistic and directive and that there is a need for additional research to guide health care providers in effectively promoting and increasing patient involvement in care [28,29]. At the same time, nurses are acutely aware of the importance of research evidence to guide nursing practice. Fortunately, research on SDT provides evidence that supporting patients' needs for autonomy, competence, and relatedness promotes behavior change in multiple primary and secondary prevention areas. These areas include diabetes self-care, substance misuse programs, weight loss, and long-term medication adherence.

In a longitudinal study among voluntary participants with diabetes, change in perceived autonomy support and change in perceived competence predicted improvement in glycemic control (hemoglobin A1c [HbA1c]) over a 12-month period. Structural equation modeling (SEM) revealed significant paths from autonomy to competence and from competence to diet, exercise, and glucose testing as well as from those activities to relative HbA1c levels. During this study, the participants saw an endocrinologist, "a nurse educator," and a registered dietician. Unfortunately, no information is provided regarding the amount of time spent with these health care providers or the content or quality of these interactions [30].

In the first clinical trial to test an SDT intervention for smoking cessation and compare its effectiveness with the community standard of care, clients in the intervention group perceived greater autonomy support and reported greater autonomy and competence than control group members. Perceptions of increased autonomy and competence also led to greater use of cessation medications and 6-month abstinence from tobacco [31]. In another study, perceived autonomy support and internal motivation predicted better methadone treatment adherence. Treatment outcomes were poor for clients who had higher levels of external motivation and low levels of internal motivation, however [32].

It is widely reported that weigh loss programs generally achieve success in the short term but that long-term weight loss and maintenance successes are elusive. In a correlational study based on SDT, participants' self-reported autonomy support and autonomy orientation were positively associated with program attendance, weight loss, and weight maintenance for nearly 24 months [33]. In other studies, long-term adherence to medications is associated with increased levels of autonomy support and autonomous motivation [34–36]. Based on this evidence, effective strategies for motivating clients to adopt and maintain healthy behaviors must be client centered and autonomy supportive.

Motivational interviewing, a counseling style based on the principles of SDT, also provides clues for outlining effective strategies. Motivational interviewing is a client-centered and directive method for enhancing clients' autonomous motivation to change by assisting them to identify and resolve ambivalence. In motivational interviewing, counselors behave in a nonjudgmental and supportive way to promote client self-exploration. Counselors accept ambivalence and resistance as normal and avoid confrontation and arguments. Clients are encouraged to discuss their behaviors so as to develop increased awareness of the discrepancies between their current behaviors and their goals and to consider alternatives. Finally, in motivational interviewing, clients need to feel competent and must feel that they have the resources and abilities to change their behavior [37,38]. The last section of this article describes strategies that nurses and other health care professionals can use in promoting clients' motivation for behavior change.

Ten strategies for nurses to use in motivating behavior change

The following list of strategies is not intended to be a "cookbook approach" or a "recipe for success" in motivating behavioral change. The factors involved in self-motivation are complex, and many are still under investigation. Based on research about SDT in practice, however, the following strategies can increase the likelihood of clients adopting and maintaining lifelong healthy behaviors (Table 1):

1. Autonomy-supportive behaviors can be learned and routinely practiced by nurses and other health care professionals working with clients across multiple health care settings. Autonomy support has been used successfully by teachers, parents, managers, and health care providers for many years [15].

2. Understand that responsibility for behavior change is like a tennis ball that is in the client's court. Clients decide whether or not to change. Nurses do not have the responsibility to decide for them [38]. Knowing this actually makes your role as a nurse easier. Your job is to understand, support, and guide the client in making a decision to adopt and sustain a healthier lifestyle. It is then for the client to choose and act.

3. Avoid trying to coerce, persuade, or reward the client. Rewards and punishments can produce amotivation or active resistance. Occasionally, rewards and punishments may bring about transient behavior changes; however, research shows that they are not associated with long-term behavior change [15].

4. Expect conflicting motivations while the client works through the process of resolving the discrepancy between his or her present situation and goals. After all, if the client was not ambivalent, he or she would not require your assistance [38].

5. Support the client's needs for relatedness by displaying a sincere interest in him or her as a unique human being who deserves your respect. The optimal nurse-client relationship for engendering autonomy support is

a type of partnership in which power is shared equally and one is not more powerful than the other [15]. Use therapeutic communication techniques to establish and maintain a nonjudgmental and empathic partnership in which the client feels safe to explore and express feelings, goals, and ambivalence, for example. Use verbal techniques, such as active listening, silence, reflection, seeking clarification, suggesting, and focusing. Ensure that kinetics and paralinguistic cues match your verbal communication [37,39].

6. Attempt to elicit "change talk." Change talk refers to client statements indicating a need for change, an intention to change, a concern with their situation, ability to change, and a notion that change is possible [38]. Clients who feel effective or competent to make a behavioral change, in addition to feeling autonomous, are more likely to be successful [15].

7. Offer information that the client may not be aware of, but do not attempt to coerce the client with threatening information. Tailor teaching-learning strategies based on the client's individual needs and culture. Offer a variety of strategies, and allow the client to determine his or her learning environment and method. Invite clients to discuss their choices, learning, and therapeutic progress with you by letting them know that you are available for such discussions.

8. Support the client's autonomy by facilitating client determination of alternatives. Offer alternatives that the client may not be aware of, and facilitate free choice among those alternatives. Allow the client to set the agenda, to decide what behavior to change, and how and when to change it. Research clearly demonstrates that clients' perceptions of autonomy support are predictive of persistent behavior change [17,33].

9. Be patient. Individuals learn, develop, and change at different rates, and one time line does not fit all. Remember that the client is (and must be) in control of the time line.

10. Provide "wise feedback" to the client. Wise feedback emphasizes the importance of several effective strategies. It involves giving explicit detail in response to the client's performance, emphasizing high standards, and communicating a belief that the client is capable of changing and maintaining the desired behavior [40]. When giving feedback, it is important to minimize or eliminate the use of controlling language because that undermines intrinsic motivation [15].

Summary

Effective nursing practice must be guided by research evidence. This article presented evidence for the application of SDT to promoting healthy behavior change in clients. The evidence is clear. When nurses and other health care providers act in ways that support clients' innate needs for autonomy, competence, and relatedness, clients are more successful at internalizing self-regulation and more inclined to adopt and maintain life-long behavioral changes. At a time when chronic illness exacts a terrible human toll and threatens to steal prosperity from future generations, it is imperative that nurses and other health care providers adopt alternative strategies for motivating their clients to live healthier lives. It is time to look to new paradigms for answers to the health care dilemmas facing our nation.

Acknowledgments

The author is thankful for the extrinsic motivation and suggestions of Karl Wheatley, PhD, in writing a paper that this article is based on. She also thanks Rosemary Sutton, PhD, for her support in her doctoral education and for teaching her the importance of giving "wise feedback" to her students. Last but not least, the author thanks Noreen Frisch, RN, PhD, FAAN, for her mentorship and for providing opportunities in nursing scholarship that she never imagined were possible.

References

[1] American Nurses Association (ANA). Nursing's social policy statement. 2nd edition. Washington, DC: American Nurse's Association; 2005.

[2] Bastable SB. Nurse as educator: principles of teaching and learning. Sudbury (MA): Jones & Bartlett; 1997.

[3] Gessner BA. Adult education: the cornerstone of patient teaching. Nurs Clin North Am 1989;24(3):589–95.

[4] Luker K, Caress A. Rethinking patient education. J Adv Nurs 1989;14(3):711–8.

[5] Hill MN, Miller NH. Compliance enhancement: a call for multidisciplinary team approaches. Circulation 1996;93:4–6.

[6] Bandura A. The primacy of self-regulation in health promotion. Applied Psychology: An International Review 2005;54(2):245–54.

[7] American Heart Association (AHA). Heart disease and stroke statistics: 2006 update. Available at: http://www.americanheart.org/downloadable/heart/1140534985281Statsupdate06book.pdf. Accessed June 18, 2006.

[8] American Heart Association. (AHA). Third report of the National Cholesterol Education Program (NCEP) Expert Panel on Detection, Evaluation, and Treatment of High Blood Cholesterol in Adults (Adult Treatment Panel III) final report. Circulation 2002;106: 3143–421.

[9] Kavey REW, Daniels SR, Lauer RM, et al. American Heart Association guidelines for primary prevention of atherosclerotic cardiovascular disease beginning in childhood. Circulation 2003;107:1562–6.

[10] Pearson TA, Blair SN, Daniels SR, et al. AHA guidelines for primary prevention of cardiovascular disease and stroke, 2002 update: consensus panel guide to comprehensive risk reduction for adult patients without coronary or other atherosclerotic vascular diseases. Circulation 2002;106:388–91.

[11] Stampfer MJ, Hu FB, Manson JE. Primary prevention of coronary heart disease in women through diet and lifestyle. N Engl J Med 2000;343:16–22.

[12] MRFIT - Multiple Risk Factor Intervention Trial Research Group. Multiple Risk Factor Intervention Trial: risk factor changes and mortality results. JAMA 1982;248(12):1465–77.

[13] HDFP - Hypertension Detection and Follow-Up Program Cooperative Group. Five year findings of the Hypertension Detection and Follow-Up Program: reduction in mortality of persons with high blood pressure, including mild hypertension. JAMA 1979;242(23): 2562–71.

[14] SHEP Cooperative Research Group. Prevention of stroke by antihypertensive drug treatment in older persons with isolated systolic hypertension. Final results of the Systolic Hypertension in the Elderly Program (SHEP). JAMA 1991;265(24):3255–64.

[15] Deci EL. Why we do what we do: understanding self-motivation. New York: Penguin; 1995.

[16] Deci EL, Ryan RM. The "what" and "why" of goal pursuits: human needs and self-determination of behavior. Psychol Inq 2000;11(4):227–68.

[17] Ryan RM, Deci EL. Self-determination theory and the facilitation of intrinsic motivation, social development, and well-being. Am Psychol 2000;55(1):68–78.

[18] Shakespeare W. Hamlet. Available at: http://www.enotes.com. Accessed June 19, 2006.

[19] Bandura A. Social foundations of thought and action: a social-cognitive theory. Englewood Cliffs (NJ): Prentice Hall; 1986.

[20] Senecal C, Nouwen A, White D. Motivation and dietary self-care in adults with diabetes: are self-efficacy and autonomous self-regulation complementary or competing constructs? Health Psychol 2000;19(5):452–7.

[21] Nigg CR, Allegrante JP, Ory M. Theory-comparison and multiple behavior research: common themes advancing health behavior research. Health Educ Res 2002;17(5):670–9.

[22] Solomon S, Kingston R. National efforts to promote behavior-change research: views from the Office of Behavioral and Social Sciences Research. Health Educ Res 2002;17(5):495–9.

[23] National Institutes of Health (NIH). Behavior Change Consortium's summary report. Available at: http://www1.od.nih.gov/behaviorchange/summary/summary.htm. Accessed October 15, 2006.

[24] Ory MG, Jordan PJ, Bazzarre T. The Behavior Change Consortium: setting the stage for a new century of health behavior change research. Health Educ Res 2002;17(5):500–11.

[25] Ferguson RF. Addressing racial disparities in high-achieving suburban schools. In: NCREL policy issues. December 2002;13:1–11. Available at: http://www.ncrel.org/policy/pubs/html/ pivot13.pdf. Accessed September 13, 2004.

[26] Sheldon KA, Williams G, Joiner T. Self-determination theory in the clinic: motivating physical and mental health. New Haven (CT): Yale University Press; 2003.

[27] Eisenberger R, Cameron J. Detrimental effects of reward: reality or myth? Am Psychol 1996; 51:1153–66.

[28] Epstein RM, Alper BS, Quill TE. Communicating evidence for participatory decision making. JAMA 2004;291(19):2359–66.

[29] Quill TE, Brody H. Physician recommendations and patient autonomy: finding a balance between physician power and patient choice. Ann Intern Med 1996;125(9):763–9.

[30] Williams GC, McGregor HA, Zeldman A, et al. Testing a self-determination theory process model for promoting glycemic control through diabetes self-management. Health Psychol 2004;23(1):58–66.

[31] Williams GC, McGregor HA, Levesque C, et al. Testing a self-determination theory intervention for motivating tobacco cessation: supporting autonomy and competence in a clinical trial. Health Psychol 2006;25(1):91–101.

[32] Zeldman A, Ryan RM. Motivation, autonomy support, and entity beliefs: their role in methadone maintenance treatment. J Soc Clin Psychol 2004;23(5):675–96.

[33] Williams GC, Grow VM, Freedman ZR, et al. Motivational predictors of weigh loss and weight-loss maintenance. J Pers Soc Psychol 1996;70(1):115–26.

[34] Kennedy S, Goggin K, Nollen N. Adherence to HIV medications: utility of the theory of self-determination. Cognit Ther Res 2004;28(5):611–28.

[35] Williams GC, Frankel RM, Campbell TL, et al. Research on relationship centered care and healthcare outcomes from the Rochester Biopsychosocial Program: a self-determination theory integration. Fam Syst Health 2000;18(1):79–90.

[36] Williams GC, Rodin GC, Ryan RM, et al. Autonomous regulation and long-term medication adherence in adult outpatients. Health Psychol 1998;17(3):269–76.

[37] Hecht J, Borrelli B, Breger RKR, et al. Motivational interviewing in community-based research: experiences from the field. Ann Behav Med 2005;29(2):29–34.

[38] Markland D, Ryan RM, Tobin VJ, et al. Motivational interviewing and self-determination theory. J Soc Clin Psychol 2005;24(6):813–31.

[39] Frisch NC, Johnson VD. Tools of psychiatric metal health nursing: communication, nursing process, and the nurse client relationship. In: Frisch NC, Frisch LE, editors. Psychiatric mental health nursing. 3rd edition. Clifton Park (NY): Thompson Delmar; 2006. p. 88–103.

[40] Cohen GL, Steele CM, Ross LD. The mentor's dilemma: providing critical feedback across the racial divide. Pers Soc Psychol Bull 1999;25(10):1302–18.

NURSING
CLINICS
OF NORTH AMERICA

Nurs Clin N Am 42 (2007) 243–259

Energy-Based Modalities

Joan Engebretson, DrPH, AHN-BC, RN[a,*],
Diane Wind Wardell, PhD, RNC[b]

[a]Department of Target Populations, School of Nursing, University of Texas Health Science
Center–Houston, 6901 Bertner Avenue, Room 764, Houston, TX 77030, USA
[b]Department of Target Populations, School of Nursing, University of Texas Health Science
Center–Houston, 6901 Bertner Avenue, Room 793, Houston, TX 77030, USA

Touch therapies and research perspectives

Human touch or laying-on of hands for the purpose of healing has been used historically and cross-culturally for centuries. Nursing has been in the lead of contemporary health care professions in recognizing the influence of touch therapies and has done so for more than 30 years. Only recently has this approach to healing been the topic of study and research in conventional medical science, however.

Touch therapies is an overall term that includes any type of use of the human hand for healing, and such therapies are generally classified as spiritual healing in the United Kingdom and Europe (E. Ernst, personal communication, 2003). In the United States, touch therapies are classified as energy therapies under the subset of biofield modalities by the National Center for Complementary and Alternative Medicine (NCCAM), which was formed in 1998 by the National Institutes of Health (NIH) [1]. Therapeutic Touch (TT), Healing Touch (HT), and Reiki as well as other spiritual or energy practices using human touch or distant healing are included in this category. These modalities have been historically described as using a vital force, which is referred to as "chi or qi" and "prana" in Eastern traditions.

The most common contemporary touch therapies used in nursing are TT, HT, and Reiki. Because a complete systematic review of research on all touch therapies and of each of these therapies is beyond the scope of this article, research is reviewed according to the most common research approaches, with examples of specific studies from these three modalities. State of science and challenges to classic research design are discussed, along with

---

* Corresponding author.
E-mail address: joan.c.engebretson@uth.tmc.edu (J. Engebretson).

0029-6465/07/$ - see front matter © 2007 Elsevier Inc. All rights reserved.
doi:10.1016/j.cnur.2007.02.004
nursing.theclinics.com

the theoretic development of the concepts related to energy healing and touch therapies.

Holistic nursing practice with touch therapies

Consistent with the nursing paradigm, touch therapies incorporate a holistic philosophy that approaches the individual within a context and ascribes a dynamic interconnectedness of multiple aspects of an individual's life and environment [2]. One of the reasons why the acceptance of these therapies in health care has been challenged is that this view is in contrast to typical Western biomedical practices, which tend to focus on specific diseases and the mechanisms of those diseases, with an the intent to cure, repair, or modify the course of the disease. Traditional biomedical approaches examine the mechanisms of function and view disease as a disruption, and they seek to treat or repair that dysfunction. This perspective is reductionistic, leading to a linear focus on parts of an individual and a view of that person's symptoms independent of the whole. These approaches are not well suited to the study of touch therapies, which is oriented to individualized holistic responses and the promotion of health. From the biomedical perspective, the argument is often offered that energy-based therapies and spiritual practices are unscientific.

Even so, public interest as well as the popularity of TT and HT in the nursing profession has spurred research in this area. Eisenberg and colleagues [3] conducted one of the initial surveys on the use of complementary and alternative medicine (CAM), of which touch therapies were included, with more than 1500 respondents and found that more than 33% used 1 or more of the 16 modalities on the questionnaire, spending more money than they did on primary care, and that nearly three fourths of them did not reveal this use to their physician. This survey was repeated 7 years later and determined that participation had increased to 42% [4]. The prevalence of energy healing significantly increased from 1.3% to 3.8%, with an estimate of nearly 40,000 visits to providers. In a more recent large survey (N = 31,000) conducted in 2002 by the Centers for Disease Control and Prevention (CDC) and the National Center for Health Statistics (NCHS), 62% of adults had used CAM within the past 12 months [5]. Of these users, more than 1% used touch therapies. This needs to be considered in relation to the fact that only 11.8% used practitioner-based therapies. Also, *energy therapies* and *Reiki* are the terms reported, and it is unclear if TT and HT was systematically investigated. It is noteworthy, however, that of the more than 300 identified CAM therapies, touch therapies are being included in major surveys.

Research into touch therapies presents unique challenges to health research. To understand the state of the science in touch therapies better, examples of specific studies are included for illustration. TT and HT are foundational to nursing and were initially developed by and for nurses [6,7]. Reiki, with Oriental roots, is currently in used by many nurses and in hospital settings even though it has a generic training program. All three of these approaches use a variety of hands-on techniques that are purported to facilitate balance within the body as well as in the biofield that surrounds the body. This balance is believed to promote physical, emotional, mental, and spiritual well-being. The nursing diagnosis that reflects understanding and use of biofield approaches is defined as follows: "Disturbed Energy Field: disruption in the flow of energy surrounding a person's being that results in a disharmony of the body, mind, and/or spirit" [8]. People use these therapies to promote health by preventing disease and promoting healthy aging, reducing symptoms of disease, and reducing side effects of treatment.

The discussion within the nursing profession has been supportive and pejorative ever since the inclusion of these therapies in the North American Nursing Diagnosis Association (NANDA) [9,10], and since their use has become more popular, the need for research and a better understanding of these modalities is recognized. It is imperative that the nursing profession remains cognizant of the importance of these therapies for patient care and to recognize the strengths and limitations of their use. Approaches to evidence-based practice should include a variety of understandings from quantitative and qualitative perspectives [11].

Research and evidence for touch therapies

One way to explore the research and evidence accumulated around touch therapies is to review studies from the perspective of the type of design that was used to research the therapy. Designs typically used in traditional health research can be broadly classified as observational and experimental.

Much research on CAM has begun with observational studies. Observational designs can be quantitative or qualitative, but all have in common the fact that they do not manipulate an independent variable. For example, epidemiologic studies can determine prevalence of the use of touch therapies or can compare two groups or study a group over a period of time without exposing them to a controlled treatment. These studies attempt to determine if there is a relation between some behavior (ie, practice of a CAM modality) and a health outcome. Qualitative approaches attempt to understand a phenomenon better within the context of a particular setting or condition. This is an appropriate approach when the phenomenon is not well understood.

Experimental designs or clinical trials are the most common designs in health care research, particularly when examining a treatment modality. Experimental designs seek to determine a cause-effect relation between the treatment (touch therapy) and a designated outcome. Meta-analytic designs systematically combine data from several existing quantitative studies to make inferences that are more generalizable. Generalized or systematic reviews do not use any type of analysis and can only provide a summary of current state of the research knowledge. Mixed method designs combine qualitative and quantitative methods in an attempt to compensate for the inherent limitations in either design. This provides a broader perspective on the issue. Currently, however, research on touch therapies presents unique challenges.

Observational approaches

People are studied in natural settings in observational studies. Surveys are one example in which the researcher might ask the participant several questions regarding behaviors, thoughts, or attitudes about a particular topic. Surveys can describe the prevalence of certain behaviors or perceptions, whereas other observational studies may retrospectively or prospectively examine a group with a certain type of behavior or compare two groups with different practices.

Surveys

Surveys have established the widespread use of CAM therapies and the increased use over time [3,4]. These and other studies [12] used time trend analysis, determined that CAM use is a secular trend that has been active at least since the 1960s, and concluded that CAM use is not a passing fad or likely to fade anytime soon.

Other surveys have focused on healers to understand better what they perceived as the effects of CAM modalities. One example of this type of study involved a large survey of CAM providers, investigating the conditions that these providers thought would benefit most from specific therapies [13]. The most common conditions these CAM providers identified were stress or anxiety, headaches, back pain, respiratory problems, insomnia, cardiovascular problems, and musculoskeletal problems. HT surveys have been conducted within hospital settings and have determined high patient satisfaction and reduction in symptoms, such as pain and anxiety [14].

Comparison observational studies

In a study of more than 2000 adults with diabetes, researchers compared a group within the sample who used CAM, including touch therapies, with other nonusers on the outcome of practicing other medical preventive behaviors, such as getting immunizations [15]. CAM users were more likely to get immunizations and other preventive care. This study demonstrated that CAM users generally do not avoid biomedicine and that CAM use is complementary to biomedicine rather than an alternative.

Case studies

Case studies provide a detailed description of individual experiences or processes, including description of the healer's experience. A detailed account of the techniques used and the longitudinal experiences of the patient can provide valuable insight into the use of techniques that are not well explored or documented.

Although many case studies are published in newsletters and nonscientific media, some detailed case studies are published in professional journals. These case studies can provide valuable understanding about touch therapies. Examples from professional citations include the use of TT with a patient experiencing pain and anxiety [16], measurement of the biofield with acupoints in a client with back pain during an HT treatment [17], and successful natural conception in a client with infertility [18].

Qualitative designs

Qualitative designs, commonly used in social sciences, focus on understanding rather than on experimentation or determining cause and effect. This design has been used with healers and recipients to help create a greater understanding of the experience and process of receiving or providing touch therapy.

Several studies have explored the experience of receiving touch therapy. For example, in one study, recipients of TT reported feeling relaxed, along with cognitive, emotional, and physical sensations as well as spiritual or transcendent experiences [19]. Several studies using HT have focused on women during cancer treatment [20–22]. These studies revealed a distinct pattern of interactions that included caring for each other; opening into trust, receptibility, and intuition; and cocreating with each other and themselves so that there was a sense of being-one-with and bonding. Further, a change in consciousness allowed participants to see themselves as whole, unified (body-emotion-mind-spirit), and having a sense of well-being.

An ethnographic study of community-based healers using Reiki and other touch therapies illuminated the centrality of spirituality to the healing work. In addition to feelings of heat, relaxation, and strong emotions, healers and recipients vividly described extraordinary spiritual experiences [23,24]. Independently reported descriptions of images and experiences were often shared by the healer and recipient.

Concerns with observational studies

One of the major concerns with survey research is that surveys generally underestimate use because they can only document the modalities on the instrument that is studied. Additionally, there may be sampling bias; even though participants may be randomly selected, the final sample often omits pockets of people who do not have or do not answer telephones or follow-up on surveys. Additionally, many of these observational studies often look at combinations of CAM, which may lump touch therapies with other CAM practices. This likely reflects common practice, because many people often use a variety of CAM or health-promoting activities. Nevertheless, the combinations can be great confounders in comparison studies. Qualitative studies are local and not designed for generalization; however, findings are often applicable to other situations.

Clinical trials and experimental designs

Experimental research or clinical trials are the most common and respected designs in biomedicine to assess the efficacy of a specific treatment. These designs expose subjects to a treatment, such as TT, HT, or Reiki, and then systematically examine a specific outcome to determine the effects of that treatment. Generally, such a group of subjects would be compared with a similar group without the treatment. In other studies, before and after comparisons are made using the subjects as their own control. These approaches generally rely on a theoretic framework to establish the outcome that is to be examined, thus providing a hypothesis to test.

Animal and laboratory models of touch therapies or energy healing

Often, new medical treatments (ie, pharmaceutics) go through a process of laboratory and animal testing; once efficacy and safety are established, the research progresses to use with human subjects. Most touch therapy research (historically considered safe by virtue of long-standing use around the world) has been conducted on humans, bypassing animal or laboratory studies. Some recent clinical trials on plant and cell lines have been conducted to help establish the physiologic mechanism of action, however.

Some examples include a study on the effect of TT on blood hemoglobin and hematocrit levels, in which it was found that after three session of TT in individuals with hemoglobin levels less than 12 g/dL, there was a significant increase in both parameters [25].

In a Reiki study, exposed bacteria showed improved growth over nonexposed bacteria [26]. These results were statistically significant for those Reiki healers in a healing context (providing Reiki to a human patient directly before an application of Reiki on the bacteria). A correlation between the general well-being of the provider and the bacterial growth was also noted. In a small study with rats, application of Reiki significantly reduced noise-induced microvascular leakage [27].

Randomized controlled trials

The randomized controlled trial (RCT) remains the "gold standard" in medical research and is the model used for most pharmaceutic and other intervention studies. Key characteristics of this design are to (1) manipulate or apply a standardized treatment (independent variable) or intervention, such as a form of touch therapy; (2) measure the impact of the treatment on predetermined outcomes; (3) design the study to control for other variables that might have an effect on an outcome; and (4) establish a causal statistical relation between the treatment and the outcome. Participants are randomly assigned to an experimental group (one receiving a standardized form of the touch therapy) and a control group (one not receiving any treatment, receiving standard care, or receiving an intervention that is used to provide the participant with additional attention that they would receive if in the experimental group). Randomization reportedly evenly distributes intervening or confounding variables across the groups. Ideally, a process of blinding is used so that neither the participants nor the investigators know who is getting the experimental intervention. This design works well in pharmaceutic studies when the control group can receive a placebo that has no active properties; however, this is much more difficult in studies of touch therapies. Attempting to blind touch therapy studies is fraught with problems; for example, participants would know if someone was touching them, and it is difficult for practitioners to "turn off" healing intentions. Using a sham healer for the control group has also been problematic, because some people are natural healers [28].

A standardized outcome measure based on the hypothesized outcome that the treatment was designed to produce is applied to both groups, or after the intervention in a single-group design. Statistical analysis is conducted to determine if the effect would be attributable to chance or to the intervention.

A blind RCT study was conducted to determine the effectiveness of TT for use with patients with dementia [29]. The findings were significant for overall score of behavioral symptoms before and after treatment in the TT group compared with the placebo and control groups. It was concluded that TT was found to be more effective than the controls in decreasing behavioral symptoms of dementia. In another blind RCT using HT as the intervention, participants undergoing treatment for gynecologic cancer had reported significant improvements in quality of life for those in the HT group compared with the control group, even though most participants believed themselves to be in the intervention group [30].

A Reiki study using an RCT design with patients who had had strokes measured the outcomes of depression and functional recovery [31]. Although no statistically significant differences were found between groups overall on the overall outcomes, the researchers did note a marked increase in a subscale of "being able to get going" in both Reiki groups. This finding suggests that Reiki might have a selective effect on mood and energy levels, but this effect did not carry over to the overall measure of depressive symptoms. Because research is in its infancy and mechanisms not are well understood, this example illustrates how an important outcome may have been missed.

Quasiexperimental designs

The major difference between true experimental and quasiexperimental designs is the lack of randomization or the absence of a control group. This may happen when one is working with small sample sizes because of resource allocation or timing. Examples are a one-group design with outcome variables measured before and after treatment or a two-group design without random assignment into groups. The treatment might be a one-time session or involve a series of sessions. Most clinical trials in touch therapies have used a quasiexperimental design.

TT has been the leader in the area of quasiexperimental designs and has accumulated a large enough body of evidence to conduct formalized analyses (see section on meta-analyses). Earlier studies reported efficacy in the following areas: reducing anxiety [32–37] and muscle relaxation and stress reduction [33,38–40].

Studies have also identified biobehavioral effects of TT. Physiologic (pulse amplitude, blood pressure, pulse, and temperature) as well as subjective measures (stress and self-assessment of health and time perception) have been examined [41]. In this study, physiologic findings of vasoconstriction rather than vasodilation indicated a state of arousal rather than relaxation.

Physiologic and behavioral aspects of healing have been studied in HT. Some examples include an increase in mobility after total knee replacement [42], a decrease in acute or chronic pain [28,43–50], improved mood and decreased anxiety or tension [47,51,52], and improved behavior [53,54].

Reiki significantly reduced pain when used as an adjuvant to opioid therapy in the management of pain [55]. In a second study, two groups were compared: one with standard opioid treatment plus rest and another receiving the same opioid treatment plus 1.5 hours of Reiki on days 1 and 4 of the study [56]. This allowed the researchers to determine if the response was attributable to Reiki rather than to rest. Their findings again revealed that those receiving Reiki reported improved pain control and improved quality of life compared with the control group.

Because previous studies on Reiki have often shown outcomes indicating relaxation, one study specifically examined autonomic nervous system changes during Reiki treatment [57]. In this study with two control groups (Reiki treatment, no treatment, and non-Reiki person mimicking Reiki hand positions), heart rate and diastolic blood pressure dropped significantly more in the Reiki group than in either of the control groups, indicating that Reiki may have an effect on the autonomic nervous system.

Limitations with using biomedical research approaches with touch therapies

Applying traditional biomedical research methods to touch therapies introduces several concerns. Touch therapies are not designed as treatments for specific diseases; appropriate outcomes, effective dosages, and time lines to detect efficacy are unknown. Many other variables, including attributes of healers, may influence potential outcomes; therefore, it is challenging to design studies that can adequately control variables so that a causal relation can be detected.

Outcome of touch therapies are often not disease specific. Biomedical research generally develops a specific treatment aimed at a specific problem based on an understanding of the mechanisms of action, which could be physical, biochemical, neurologic, or genetic. Understanding of the mechanism of disease or disorder is critical to matching an intervention to alter the progress of disease, restore function to an organ or system, or repair a malfunctioning aspect.

Touch therapies are used to restore balance in people with different diagnoses or health conditions and are understood to operate on an individual level; thus, the action may be different with each treatment. Therefore, finding a good outcome measure to examine the effectiveness over a group of people is difficult. For example, one person might find that a specific touch therapy reduced pain, another might get better sleep, and a third might have lower anxiety or blood pressure. Hence, measuring blood pressure in a person with normal blood pressure would not show any result, whereas not measuring sleep might miss a therapeutic effect. Additionally, these therapies are often used to promote health or even prevent disease. In this case, research outcomes are difficult to determine because the averted outcome is basically unknown.

Establishing an appropriate time to detect effect is variable or unknown. Another challenge is establishing an appropriate time frame in which to determine the effect, because the time period may not be known or, more often, may be variable. For example, one person may experience some effects immediately, whereas others may not experience the effects for a day or more; thus, even a well-designed study may miss the salient effect. Because touch therapies may be based on subtle energies, larger groups and longer treatment periods may be needed [58,59].

Appropriate dosage is unknown. Appropriate dosage is a critical element in assessing the efficacy of treatment. How much "energy healing" (ie, one session or a series) the person should have to observe an effect is not well established. There is no established protocol for any of the touch modalities. The amount of time is often determined by the healer's sense of adequacy or study design. This may be determined in the length of time per session or the number of sessions and may vary among healers or between individual patients or even within a single patient related to his or her condition.

Establishing adequate controls is difficult. One of the largest confounders of establishing a causal relation for a treatment is the placebo effect, or the healing effects of a belief in the therapy. One HT study sought to answer the question of placebo effect by evaluating predictor questions about beliefs, expectations, and behaviors and found no difference in the responders and nonresponders related to treatment effects [60].

There may be variation in the preparation or innate characteristics of healers. Standardization of the treatment is essential in biomedical research.

Variation in the healer may be a confounding variable. TT and HT have curricula of study and certification of their practitioners in an attempt to standardize the qualifications of their practitioners. Reiki has a common initiation; however, the preparation of the healer may vary from a weekend workshop to a close lengthy apprenticeship with a Reiki master. Regardless of the training, the question remains whether the effect is attributable to the modality or to the skills of an individual healer. Some studies have suggested that more experienced healers have better outcomes [60,61].

Mixed methods

Mixed methods, a combination of qualitative and quantitative strategies, used sequentially or combined within the same study, is an emerging design that can help to overcome the limitations of each method separately. In one example, an HT study examining quality of life at the end stage of life used an experimental design along with qualitative interviews [62]. There were no significant differences between those who had received standard hospice care and those who received HT along with hospice care; however, interpersonal, well-being, and function scores showed improvement in the HT group over time as compared with the control group, in which these variables declined. The qualitative findings reported by the participants described experiences that helped to demonstrate the complex nature of the experience as reported by this participant [62]:

> ... I don't know why things are the way they are or why I feel the way I do about it, because I was really very skeptical about it. If anybody can be relaxed for a couple of hours, then it is wonderful ... Even a couple of hours it is wonderful to be relaxed. It lasts longer than that, probably 2–4 hours. Actually, it goes on longer—it just doesn't stop. The next day even and the next day ...

A nonrandomized two-group design of HT and progressive muscle relaxation was used in 12 veterans experiencing chronic neuropathic pain. This study reported that HT might have some effects on altering the pain experience in these veterans, although there was large variation within the groups. The qualitative analysis helped to inform the study by describing the varied experiences of the participants, including absence of pain after treatment, relief attributed to other factors, and no relief experienced [63].

Wardell and Engebretson [64] integrated a qualitative interview and observations during the treatment in a quasiexperimental design. This study examined physiologic and biochemical effects of a single 30-minute Reiki treatment. State or trait anxiety, salivary IgA, and cortisol were measured before and after the Reiki treatment. Blood pressure and biofeedback measures were taken at intervals before, during, and after the treatment. Participants were interviewed after the Reiki treatment. Comparing before and after measures, anxiety was significantly reduced and salivary IgA levels rose. These findings suggest that Reiki may increase relaxation, decrease anxiety, and increase humoral immunologic function. During the interviews, participants reported a liminal state of awareness (changes in orientation to time) as well as paradoxical sensate and symbolic experiences [65]. These paradoxical findings, also indicative of an altered state of consciousness, suggest that many linear models commonly used in medical research may be inappropriate to capture the experience of recipients of touch therapies. This study established potential biologic parameters and contributed to the development of theoretic frameworks for future studies.

Meta-analytic approaches and systematic reviews

Meta-analysis is used when there is enough completed research to support combining the findings from several studies to provide a more convincing argument for the interpretation of these findings. Only TT has had enough published studies in which meta-analyses could be conducted. Two studies have found a moderate effect size for positive results on psychologic and physiologic variables hypothesized to be influenced by TT [66,67]. These were primarily the reduction of anxiety and pain. There were, however, mixed or negative results in some of the studies included in the analyses, because biomedical research also looks at the accumulation of evidence on which to base conclusions. A process of conducting systematic reviews can be used to look at the accumulation of evidence. One study systematically reviewed touch healing research, primarily on TT, in 19 RCTs involving 1122 patients; of these, 11 (58%) studies reported statistically significant treatment effects [68]. Another systematic review of all studies that used an experimental or quasiexperimental design on the efficacy of TT on wound healing was conducted [69]. In the 4 studies that met the criteria, the effects were variable, with 2 studies demonstrating a significant effect of TT, whereas the other 2 trials did not show an effect. Thus, the conclusion is that there is insufficient evidence that TT promotes wound healing.

More than 30 studies of HT were reviewed, and the authors found encouraging results for pain management as well as subjective benefits in mood, well-being, and interpersonal relationships in patients with cancer [70]. Patients with cancer also had an increase in vitality. Several positive outcomes related to well-being, spirituality, and functional status were reported in studies of HT in the elderly.

According to another review of touch therapies, some of the outcomes that have been examined along this line are pain, mood, anxiety, relaxation, functional status, health status, well-being, wound healing, blood pressure, and immune function [71]. Although there is support for this, some studies are more equivocal.

Theoretic development

Although there have been considerable investigation and speculation about touch therapies, there are no well-developed theories that would establish a solid base for traditional research. Wilber [59] has developed a taxonomy of subtle energies that draws on some of the world's great wisdom traditions, many which practice forms of touch for healing. This model or theory is the beginning of integrating and classifying these world views of healing into a unified language necessary for theoretic development.

Much of the current research on touch therapies has applied a theory of psychoneuroimmunologic hypothesizing that touch therapies evoke the parasympathetic response in the direction of relaxation, contributing to lower anxiety, stress, and pain and increased humeral immunity as well as a sense of well-being. The mechanisms are not well established, however, and it is likely that this explanatory framework is insufficient to explain what healers and recipients describe. In some cases, findings can be paradoxical or complex. For example, some recipients have extraordinary or religious experiences and may not be in a state of psychophysiologic relaxation.

Some of the basic theoretic notions about touch therapies are that they are a form of (1) spiritual healing, thereby beyond understanding, or (2) balancing subtle energies to restore the individual to a healthier state. Neither one of these theories is readily testable. Spiritual healing posits a notion of consciousness and thought and includes distance healing. A review of distant healing that included noncontact touch therapies and other forms of distant healing, such as prayer, was conducted [72]. Statistically significant positive treatment effects were demonstrated in 57% of the 23 trials involving 2774 patients. These findings are somewhat equivocal; the entire genre of research in spiritual healing or prayer is extremely controversial, highlighting the difficulty of research in this realm, and is beyond the scope of this article. Challenging the phenomenon of energy, many of the reported effects do not dissipate with distance or are not blocked with conventional energy barriers [68].

A new approach, complexity science, is making its way into health-related research. With it base in theoretic physics, originally applied to astrophysics (macrosystems) and subatomic levels (microsystems), this scientific approach has more recently been applied to earth sciences, computers, economics, and social and organizational systems as well as, most recently, to biology and health care [73]. Hankey [74] promotes expanding the traditional biochemistry perspectives of medicine by exploring the biophysics of biologic systems to acquire a better understanding of adaptive systems.

One of the concepts of complexity science is that humans and organizations are complex adaptive systems and not reducible to linear approaches. This notion of the human as a self-organizing complex adaptive system is emerging as a new paradigm for clinical practice in the health care field [75] and may also provide a new approach to research. Walach [76] has postulated that entanglement, another concept from complexity science, may provide a solution to the question of how touch therapies, nonlocal healing, and ritual healing may possibly work.

Rubik [77] proposes a biofield hypothesis, drawing on many constructs of complexity science. She views humans as complex, adaptive, nonlinear, dynamic, self-organizing systems with emergent properties that are constantly exchanging "energy-with-information" at multiple levels with their surroundings. She also considers medical interventions in two categories: (1) structural interactions, which describe many mainstream medical interventions, and (2) regulatory interactions, which act informationally on the organism. She posits that touch therapies are mediated by means of extremely low-level electromagnetic fields emitted by the healer's hands, which serve as antennae for elements of the biofield and are uniquely associated with psychophysiologic states of the practitioner's intention. Regulatory interactions and the impact and mechanisms of self-organization and healing have a theoretic fit with energy balance and reported changes in the autonomic nervous system. Other researchers have developed frameworks hypothesizing that bioenergy is electromagnet in nature and that its transmission, reception, and processing interface with cellular- and molecular-level events could be detectable by physical instruments or biomarkers [78]. These new vistas show much promise in the development of future research in this ancient yet not well-understood healing modality.

Summary

Research on touch therapies is still in the early stages of development. Studies of TT, HT, and Reiki are quite promising; however, at this point, they can only suggest that these healing modalities have efficacy in reducing anxiety; improving muscle relaxation; aiding in stress reduction, relaxation, and sense of well-being; promoting wound healing; and reducing pain. This is important, because chronic pain is a major problem that is likely to continue with the aging of the population. Management of chronic pain is difficult and challenging. Other research has begun to unravel the complex psychoneurobiologic mechanisms in stress, pain, and immunity. To date, there have been no serious side effects attributed to any of these healing modalities. Therefore, the clinical implications are that these modalities can be used in many situations by healers who have had training in one of the approaches to touch therapy.

Several methodologic research issues have been raised, including standardization, practitioner qualifications, and appropriateness of the measures and outcome criteria for significance. These issues are inherent when one tries to "fit" a holistic and complex process into the reductionistic scientific model. New and more appropriate methods, such as those developed in relation to complexity theory, hold promise for better understanding and more cogent research. Current NIH funding is supporting research into the physiologic basis and behavioral aspects of these energy therapies. In the future, hopefully, more definitive statements about their mechanisms of action and effects can be applied.

Nursing care is enhanced by the use of these approaches [79]. As nurses, it is important to recognize and support spiritual aspects of healing [80]. The application of complexity science to health and healing also holds much intrigue for nursing, because this approach allows for the nonlinear understanding of holistic systems. The multidimensional aspects of healing inherent in patient care continue to be expanded and facilitated by our understanding and application of energy therapies.

References

[1] NIH. National Center for Complementary and Alternative Medicine. 1998 National Institutes of Health. Available at: http://nccam.nih.gov/health/whatiscam/. Accessed October 24, 2006.

[2] Cassidy CM. Social science and theory in the study of alternative and complementary medicine. J Altern Complement Med 1994;1(1):19–40.

[3] Eisenberg DM, Kessler RC, Foster C, et al. Unconventional medicine in the United States. Prevalence, costs, and patterns of use. N Engl J Med 1993;328(4):246–52.

[4] Eisenberg DM, Davis RB, Ettner SL, et al. Trends in alternative medicine use in the United States, 1990–1997: results of a follow-up national survey. J Am Med Assoc 1998;280(18): 1569–75.

[5] Barnes PM, Powell-Griner E, McFann K, et al. Complementary and alternative medicine use among adults: United States, 2002. Adv Data 1994;27(343):1–19.

[6] Krieger D. Accepting your power to heal. Sante Fe (MN): Bear & Co; 1993.

[7] Mentgen J. Healing touch. Nurs Clin North Am 2002;36(1):143–57.

[8] NANDA. NANDA: nursing diagnoses: definitions and classification, 2005–2006. Philadelphia: NANDA International; 2005.

[9] Wardell DW. Response to letter to the editor. J Nurs Scholarsh 2004;36(3):288–9.

[10] Henkelman WJ. Letter to the editor: healing touch is pseudoscience. J Nurs Scholarsh 2004; 36(4):288.

[11] Fawcett J, Watson J, Neuman B, et al. On nursing theories and evidence. J Nurs Scholarsh 2001;33(2):115–9.

[12] Kessler RC, Davis RB, Foster DF, et al. Long-term trends in the use of complementary and alternative medical therapies in the United States. Ann Intern Med 2001;135(4):262–8.

[13] Long L, Huntley A, Ernst E. Which complementary and alternative therapies benefit which conditions? A survey of the opinions of 223 professional organizations. Complement Ther Med 2001;9(3):178–85.

[14] Wardell D. Research survey. 8th edition. Lakewood (CO): Healing Touch International, Inc; 2006.

[15] Garrow D, Egede LE. National patterns and correlates of complementary and alternative medicine use in adult patients with diabetes. J Altern Complement Med 2006;12(9):895–902.

[16] Green CA. Reflection of a therapeutic touch experience: case study 2. Complement Ther Nurs Midwifery 1998;4(1):17–21.

[17] Forbes MA, Rust R, Becker GJ. Surface electromyography (EMG) apparatus as a measurement device for biofield research: results from a single case. J Altern Complement Med 2004; 10(4):617–26.

[18] Kissinger J, Kaczmarek L. Healing touch and fertility: a case report. J Perinat Educ 2006; 15(2):13–20.

[19] Sneed NV, Olson M, Bonadonna R. The experience of therapeutic touch for novice recipients. J Holist Nurs 1997;15(3):243–53.

[20] Christiano C. The lived experience of healing touch with cancer patients [master's thesis]. Florida International University in Miami; 1997.

[21] Kopecki D. The lived experience of women with breast cancer [master's thesis]. The Sage Colleges; 2001.

[22] Mooreland K. The lived experience of receiving the chakra connection of women with breast cancer who are receiving chemotherapy: a phenomenological study. Healing Touch Newsletter 1998;8(3):3 5.

[23] Engebretson J. Comparison of nurses and alternative healers. Image J Nurs Sch 1996;28(2): 95–9.

[24] Engebretson J. Urban healers: an experiential description of American healing groups. Qual Health Res 1996;6(4):528–43.

[25] Movaffaghi Z, Hasanpoor M, Farsi M, et al. Effects of therapeutic touch on blood hemoglobin and hematocrit level. J Holist Nurs 2006;24(1):41–8.

[26] Rubik B, Brooks AJ, Schwartz GE. In vitro effect of Reiki treatment on bacterial cultures: role of experimental context and practitioner well-being. J Altern Complement Med 2006; 12(1):7–13.

[27] Baldwin AL, Schwartz GE. Personal interaction with a Reiki practitioner decreases noise-induced microvascular damage in an animal model. J Altern Complement Med 2006;12(1):15–22.

[28] Slater V. Safety, elements, and effects of healing touch on chronic non-malignant abdominal pain [unpublished doctoral dissertation]. University of Tennessee, College of Nursing, Knoxville (TN); 1996.

[29] Wood DL, Craven RF, Whitney J. The effect of therapeutic touch on behavioral symptoms of persons with dementia. Altern Ther Health Med 2005;11(1):66–74.

[30] Cook CA, Guerrerio JF, Slater VE. Healing touch and quality of life in women receiving radiation treatment for cancer: a randomized controlled trial. Altern Ther Health Med 2004; 10(3):34–41.

[31] Shiflett SC, Navak S, Bid C, et al. Effect of Reiki treatments on functional recovery in patients in poststroke rehabilitation: a pilot study. J Altern Complement Med 2002;8(6):755–63.

[32] Heidt P. The effects of therapeutic touch on anxiety level of hospitalized patients. Nurs Res 1981;30:32–7.

[33] Quinn J. Therapeutic touch as energy exchange: replication and extension. Nurs Sci Q 1989; 2(2):79–87.

[34] Ferrell-Torry A, Glick O. The use of therapeutic massage as a nursing intervention to modify anxiety and the perception of cancer pain. Cancer Nurs 1993;16:93–101.

[35] Simington J, Laing G. Effects of therapeutic touch on anxiety in the institutionalized elderly. Clin Nurs Res 1993;2:438–50.

[36] Adamat R, Killingworth A. Care of the critically ill patient: the impact of stress on the use of touch in intensive therapy units. J Adv Nurs 1994;19:912–22.

[37] Gagne D, Toye R. The effects of therapeutic touch and relaxation therapy in reducing anxiety. Arch Psychiatr Nurs 1994;8:184–9.

[38] Randolph G. Therapeutic and physical touch: physiologic response to stressful stimuli. Nurs Res 1984;33:33–6.

[39] Olson M, Sneed N, LaVia M, et al. Stress-induced immunosuppression and therapeutic touch. Altern Ther Health Med 1997;3(2):68–74.

[40] Peck SD. The effectiveness of therapeutic touch for decreasing pain in elders with degenerative arthritis. J Holist Nurs 1997;15(2):176–98.

[41] Engle VF, Graney MJ. Biobehavioral effects of therapeutic touch. J Nurs Scholarsh 2000; 32(3):287–93.

[42] Cordes P, Proffitt C, Roth J. The effect of healing touch therapy on the pain and joint mobility experienced by patients with total knee replacements. Healing Touch Research Survey, June 2002. Lakewood (CO): Healing Touch International, Inc; 2002.

[43] Darbonne M. The effect of HT modalities on patients with chronic pain [unpublished master's thesis]. Northwestern State University, Natchitoches, Louisiana; 1997.

[44] Diener D. A pilot study of the effect of chakra connection and magnetic unruffled on perception of pain in people with fibromyalgia. Healing Touch Newsletter Research Edition 2001; 01(3):7–8.

[45] Merritt P, Randall D. The effect of healing touch and other forms of energy work on cancer pain [abstract]. Healing Touch International Research Survey. Lakewood (CO): Healing Touch International, Inc; 2002.

[46] Protzman L. The effect of healing touch on pain and relaxation [abstract]. Healing Touch International Research Survey. Lakewood (CO): Healing Touch International, Inc; 2002.

[47] Post-White J, Kinney ME, Savik K, et al. Therapeutic massage and healing touch improve symptoms in cancer. Integr Cancer Ther 2003;2(4):332–44.

[48] Wardell DW. The trauma release technique: how it is taught and experienced in healing touch. Alternative & Complementary Therapies 2000;6(1):20–7.

[49] Welcher B, Kish J. Reducing pain and anxiety through healing touch. Healing Touch Newsletter 2001;01(3):19.

[50] Weymouth K, Sandberg-Lewis S. Comparing the efficacy of healing touch and chiropractic adjustment in treating chronic low back pain: a pilot study. Healing Touch Newsletter 2000; 00(3):7–8.

[51] Seskevich JE, Crater SW, Lane JD, et al. Beneficial effects of noetic therapies on mood before percutaneous intervention for unstable coronary syndromes. Nurs Res 2004;53(2):116–21.

[52] Taylor B. The effects of healing touch on the coping ability, self-esteem and general health of undergraduate nursing students. Complement Ther Nurs Midwifery February 2001;7(1): 34–42.

[53] Wang K, Hermann C. Pilot study to test the effectiveness of healing touch on agitation in people with dementia. Geriatr Nurs 2006;27(1):34–40.

[54] Verret P. Healing touch as a relaxation intervention in children with spasticity. Healing Touch Newsletter, 2000;00(3):6–7.

[55] Olson K, Hanson J. Using Reiki to manage pain: a preliminary report. Cancer Prev Control 1997;1(2):108–13.

[56] Olson K, Hanson J, Michaud M. A phase II trial of Reiki for the management of pain in advanced cancer patients. J Pain Symptom Manage 2003;26(5):990–7.

[57] Mackay N, Hansen S, McFarlane O. Autonomic nervous system changes during Reiki treatment: a preliminary study. J Altern Complement Med 2004;10(6):1077–81.

[58] Gaus W, Hogel J. Studies on the efficacy of unconventional therapies. Problems and designs. Arzneimittelforschung 1995;45(1):88–92.

[59] Wilber K. Toward a comprehensive theory of subtle energies. Explore: The Journal of Science and Healing, 2005;1(4):252–70.

[60] Wilkinson D, Knox P, Chatman J, et al. The clinical effectiveness of healing touch. J Altern Complement Med 2002;8(1):33–47.

[61] Schwartz GE, Swanick S, Sibert W, et al. Biofield detection: role of bioenergy awareness training and individual differences in absorption. J Altern Complement Med 2004;10(1): 167–9.

[62] Ziembroski J, Gilbert N, Bossarte R, et al. Healing touch and hospice care: examining outcomes at the end of life. Alternative & Complementary Therapies 2003;9(3):146–51.

[63] Wardell DW, Rintala D, Duan Z, et al. A pilot study of healing touch and progressive relaxation for chronic neuropathic pain in persons with spinal cord injury. J Holist Nurs 2006; 24(3):231–40.

[64] Wardell D, Engebretson J. Biological correlates of Reiki touch healing. J Adv Nurs 2001; 33(4):439–45.

[65] Engebretson J, Wardell D. Experience of a Reiki session. Altern Ther Health Med 2002;8(2): 48–53.

[66] Peters RM. The effectiveness of therapeutic touch: a meta-analytic review. Nurs Sci Q 1999; 12(1):52–61.

[67] Winstead-Fry P, Wijek J. An integrative review and meta-analysis of therapeutic touch research. Altern Ther Health Med 1999;5(6):58–67.

[68] Astin JA, Harkness E, Ernst E. The efficacy of "distant healing": a systematic review of randomized trials. Ann Intern Med 2000;132(11):903–10.

[69] O'Mathuna DP, Ashford RL. Cochrane Database Syst Rev 2003;(4):CD002766.

[70] Wardell DW, Weymouth K. Review of studies of healing touch. J Nurs Scholarsh 2004; 36(2):147–54.

[71] Warber SL, Gordon A, Gillespie BW, et al. Standards for conducting clinical biofield energy healing research. Altern Ther Health Med 2003;9(3 Suppl):A54–64.

[72] Jonas WB, Crawford CC. The healing presence: can it be reliably measured? J Altern Complement Med 2005;10(5):751–6.

[73] Turcotte C, Rundle JB. Self-organized complexity in the physical, biological and social sciences. Proc Natl Acad Sci U S A 2002;99(Suppl):2463–5.

[74] Hankey A. CAM modalities can stimulate advances in theoretical biology. Evid Based Complement Alternat Med 2005;2(1):5–12.

[75] Brown CA. The application of complex adaptive systems theory to clinical practice in rehabilitation. Disabil Rehabil 2006;28(9):587–93.

[76] Walach H. Generalized entanglement: a new theoretical model for understanding the effects of complementary and alternative medicine. J Altern Complement Med 2005;11(3):549–59.

[77] Rubik B. The biofield hypothesis: its biophysical basis and role in medicine. J Altern Complement Med 2002;8(6):703–17.

[78] Hintz KJ, Yount GL, Kadar I, et al. Bioenergy definitions and research guidelines. Altern Ther Health Med 2003;9(3):A13–30.

[79] Watson J, Dossey B, Dossey L. Postmodern nursing and beyond. Edinburgh (UK): Churchill Livingstone; 2000. 1999.

[80] Wardell DW, Engebretson J. Taxonomy of the spiritual experience. J Relig Health 2006; 45(2):215–33.

NURSING
CLINICS
OF NORTH AMERICA

Nurs Clin N Am 42 (2007) 261–277

Imagery in the Clinical Setting: A Tool for Healing

Terry Reed, RN, MS, HN-BC[a,b],*

[a]Beyond Ordinary Nursing, Certificate Program in Imagery, PO Box 8177, Foster City, CA 94404, USA
[b]Mills-Peninsula Health Services, Institute for Health and Healing, 100 South San Mateo Drive, San Mateo, CA 94401, USA

The use of imagery in the clinical setting exemplifies the holistic nursing model. It creates a healing relationship within the body, mind, and spirit of the patient and between the nurse and the patient. This article demonstrates through research, theory, and clinical applications the safe and successful interventions of imagery and its significant health outcomes. Case examples show how suited and vital nurses are in advancing the understanding and use of imagery, and the patient responses point the way toward bringing holistic approaches into mainstream nursing and health care in general.

History of imagery and healing

The use of imagery as an approach to support healing goes back as far as recorded history. Shamanic healing, which dates back to ancient times, used imagery in the form of prayer and ritual. In those ancient times and throughout the Dark Ages (400–1100 AD), healing and the use of imagery incorporated a mind, body, spirit, or holistic approach. During the 1600s, the Scientific Revolution and the influence of Descartes created what is commonly called the mind-body split, leading to a reductionistic view of health and healing. It is interesting to note that with the discovery of quantum physics in the 1920s, Hans Selye's work on stress in the 1940s, and current mind-body research, health care approaches are coming full circle from the focus on the physical body and "curing" to a focus on holism and "healing." Imagery is one of the many holistic approaches currently being used in nursing.

---

* Mills-Peninsula Health Services, Institute for Health and Healing, 100 South San Mateo Drive, San Mateo, CA 94401.
E-mail address: terry@integrativeimagery.com

doi:10.1016/j.cnur.2007.03.006 *nursing.theclinics.com*

What is imagery and why does it work?

If you can worry or find your parked car, you are using imagery. Just as we all dream, we use imagery to picture a scene in our mind's eye, recall a pleasant childhood memory or hear a favorite piece of music [1].

Imagery is a therapeutic process that facilitates working with the power of the imagination to affect mental attitude positively, elicit positive outcomes, and activate innate healing within the body. Unfortunately, culture has taught people to dwell more on negative emotions and events, such as worries, fears, and time pressures, so that most people have more experiences with negative rather than positive imagery. Imagery is the therapeutic tool that can be used to release stressful images, slow the racing mind, and shift the body to a peaceful place.

Imagery is a natural thought process involving the mind and the right side of the brain. The image or thought is experienced with one or more of the senses with an associated emotion linking the mind with a feeling state and the body with a resulting physiologic change. The body does not know the difference between what one is thinking and what is actually happening. As an example, an employee imagines that he or she is going to be included in an impending layoff at work. As a result, feelings of anxiety are experienced; the body responds by secreting adrenalin and cortisol, interfering with the immune system and the person's ability to cope. Where one places his or her thoughts affects his or her "inner pharmacy." A person can turn on the adrenalin or the endorphin button through the mind's eye. Imagery engages the person where that physiology begins. It is evidence based, cost-effective, noninvasive, and safe and can be used for virtually any situation from birth to death. Applications and case examples are addressed elsewhere in this article. Definitions of terms related to imagery are presented in Table 1.

Meditation is different from imagery and hypnosis in that although it is a focused state of mental concentration, it is more passive. The focal point in meditation may be the breath, a word, a phrase, or an object. The goal is not to clear the mind of all thoughts, because that is a difficult, if not impossible, goal. Rather, it is to reach a deeper level of awareness, neutrality, and inner peace. Out of this emerges wisdom and compassion for oneself and others [1].

Psychoneuroimmunology and imagery

Imagery is a perfect illustration of the mind-body connection. Before reviewing data on imagery in practice, it is prudent to describe the body of theoretic knowledge and research data that explain how and why imagery works. Psychoneuroimmunology (PNI) is a tool from which our understanding of imagery derives.

Aristotle, Darwin, and Sir William Osler (the father of modern medicine) were struck by the mind-body connection, but their only investigative tools

Table 1
Definition of terms related to imagery

Clinical hypnosis	Integrative imagery	Guided imagery
Practitioner uses suggestive language	Practitioner uses patient's words and images; facilitates interactivity with image	Scripted; sometimes suggested images are open ended
Practitioner often leads the patient to new insights	Practitioner facilitates use of patient's inner resources	Same
Induction has different levels of trance states	Induction is simple breathing and relaxation	Same
Treatment focused	Education focused	Supportive and suggestive
Real time as 1:1 approach	Real time as 1:1 approach	Compact disk, tape, or group approach

Courtesy of Beyond Ordinary Nursing; with permission. © 2003 Beyond Ordinary Nursing, Foster City, CA.

Example of integrative imagery: a patient imagines pain as a ball of fire. When the imagery practitioner asks how the patient feels about the image, the patient responds that the fireball looks threatening and scary. The imagery practitioner suggests that the patient and the fireball find a way to communicate. When asked its response to the patient, the fireball communicates that it feels scared and alone without any help. The patient is surprised and offers to help. The fireball says it did not know there was anyone who cared and becomes less red and much smaller. The patient and the fireball agree to help each other and keep in communication. The patient experiences a decrease in pain.

were dissection, microscopes, and radiographs. The science of their day was not powerful enough to discern links between the mind and the body. With the convergence of molecular biology and modern research methods, however, well-known scientists, such as Steven Locke, Carl Simmington, Richard Ader, George Soloman, Ed Blalock, and Candace Pert, presented research findings that started a paradigm shift. The shift is not so different as what occurred when the earth was thought to be at the center of the universe and that idea gave way to sun-centered theory and the discovery that the world was not flat. With the advent of neuroscience, knowledge that the central nervous system, the endocrine system, and the immune system are not separate systems but one emerged. The new paradigm is called PNI and presents a new way of thinking about the old anatomy and physiology theories. Just as in the time of Columbus, there is resistance to the new ideas and a lack of understanding about PNI, even though there has been a body of research since the 1980s.

The term *psychoneuroimmunology* was introduced by Ader and colleagues [2] in their landmark book. Ader and colleagues [2] defined PNI as "the study of interaction among behavioral, neural, endocrine and immunological processes of adaptation". Many years later, PNI is now an intense research topic that emerged in neuroscience and has now extended to influence psychology, psychiatry, endocrinology, physiology, and the biomedical community. An extensive summary of the historical advancement of PNI can be found in the article by Fleshner and Laudenslager [3]. Many nurse-scientists have also contributed a large body of research in the PNI literature [4–7]. Some of the contributions include the creation of models for further research that can guide holistic applications, such as the minimization of discomfort, prevention of disease, enhancement of coping, and overall improvement of health care.

Mind-body connection

As discussed previously, thoughts or images that elicit emotions start the cascade of biochemicals, called peptides, throughout the body-mind. As an example, a driver cuts in front of your car on the freeway, almost causing an accident. You think to yourself, "what a jerk" and feel the emotion of fear and anger. Signals by way of peptides, such as adrenalin, lead to physiologic changes, such as the fight-or-flight response, and behavioral responses, such as making angry gestures and yelling.

Peptides are biochemical substances that travel throughout the body, such as adrenalin, acetylcholine, interleukins or cytokines, insulin, angiotensin, dopamine, endorphins, and serotonin. Receptors are protein molecules that float on all cells throughout the body. The receptors are often referred to as the locks, and the peptides are the keys. The entire surface of all cells have many different receptors on them, and when they bind with their unique peptide, a disturbance is created like a key in a lock that tickles the peptide to change its shape until the chemical information enters the cell. There are as many receptors as biochemicals in the body. There have been more than 100 peptides discovered, and the number increases each year. As Pert [8], a leading neuroscientist, describes, "Peptides ooze through the body ... what keeps it all straight are the receptors throughout the body."

Pert [8] states that memory is encoded in cells at the receptor level. It is speculated that memory processes are emotionally driven and unconscious, but like other receptor-mediated processes, they can sometimes be made conscious. The notion of cellular memory is often given in presentations by clinicians who practice guided imagery. One of the teachers of this author reported a story of student nurses who were asked to imagine having boiling water spilled on their hands to see if there would be any change in the skin color. Only one nurse had such a reaction at the exact location where she actually had such an experience in childhood. This is an example of memory being held at the receptor level in the student nurse's hand; the memory was emotionally driven by the imagery state that emotionally started the biochemical flow that led to the color change in the hand. Potentially, one can retrieve different memories depending on the biochemical state, such as with the use of imagery. If the memory is traumatic, for example, reframing the experience could recreate a healing state.

Cells not only have receptor sites but secrete and store peptides. The immune system not only defends the body but makes chemicals that regulate emotions. Lymphocytes make endorphins and corticotropin. Emotions can originate in the mind and the body, and this process can happen simultaneously. Thus, not only is there ample evidence of chemical communication, but it is bidirectional. The understanding and application of PNI concepts can provide nurses with the understanding that provides a holistic approach that is preventative and promotes healing and well-being in health care. The PNI cycle in Fig. 1 created for Beyond Ordinary Nursing by faculty member

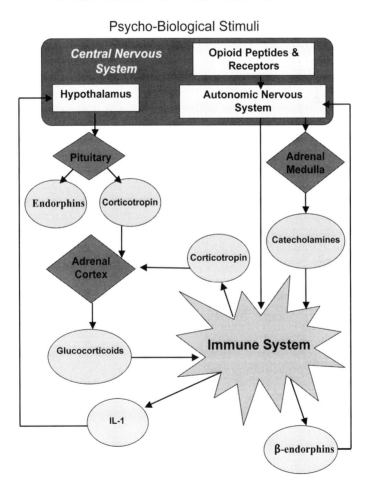

Fig. 1. PNI cycle demonstrates bidirectional flow of the opioid peptides and the interaction of receptors and peptides that demonstrates the mind-body connection. IL, interleukin. (*Adapted from* McCane KL, Huether SC. Pathophysiology: the biologic basis for disease in adults and children. 3rd edition. St. Louis (MO): Mosby; 1998; with permission.)

Guyot illustrates bidirectional flow of the opioid peptides and the interaction of receptors and peptides that demonstrates the mind-body connection.

Mind-body research in nursing

A PNI approach in nursing research is consistent with a holistic approach that takes into consideration the full spectrum of human experiences: social, economic, cultural, physical, mental, and spiritual. An excellent model of a PNI-based theoretic framework for the study of physiologic patterns that contribute to the dynamics of health has recently been published [5] and is presented in Fig. 2. The model stresses the multidimensional nature and complexity of the stress response and the role of coping strategies in altering these responses. Thanks to PNI research, perceived stress, locus of control, beliefs, and the emotions that follow demonstrate the mind-body connection, such as the impact of cortisol on the downregulation of the immune system. Incorporating the mind-body approach in research can greatly contribute to a holistic evaluation of stress-management interventions that seek to provide avenues for holistic change that can reduce perceived stress, enhance coping, and contribute to improved quality of life.

Nursing scope of practice and imagery

Imagery has the foundation of PNI to describe the how and why it works. Holistic nursing theory also provides the foundation that supports imagery as an independent nursing function. Some of the theorists that provide such a theoretic framework are M.E. Levine, Jean Watson, Margaret Newman,

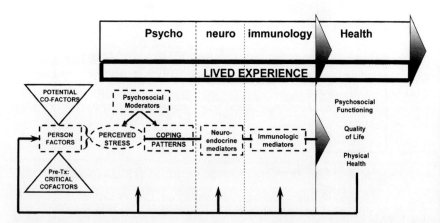

Fig. 2. PNI theoretic framework. (*From* McCain NL, Gray DP, Walter J, et al. Implementing a comprehensive approach to the study of health dynamics using the psychoneuroimmunology paradigm. Tx, treatment. ANS Adv Nurs Sci 2005;283:20–32; with permission.)

and Martha Rogers. Rogers' [9] theory on the science of unitary human beings describes humans and their environments in a dynamic interplay in which each is continually affecting and being affected by the other. In Rogers' theory, the most important conceptual feature for nursing practice is the capacity of a person to participate knowingly in the process of change [10].

Imagery as a complementary alternative medicine (CAM) modality in nursing has given rise to position statements written by many state boards of nursing and professional organizations, such as the American Holistic Nurses Association [11]. Imagery is frequently listed as an example of complementary therapies considered in the registered nurse's (RN's) scope of practice. The Nurse Practice Act identifies the practice of nursing in each state, and is therefore the primary document to delineate the use of imagery. Some of the state boards of nursing define the accepted CAM modalities but also speak to education required to perform the modality, as demonstrated in the following excerpt from the California Board of Registered Nursing [12] on CAM nursing practice.

> The competency of a registered nurse to perform the skills of CAM therapies begins with nursing education and ends with the safe nursing practice of those skills in such a way that ensures the safety, comfort, personal hygiene, and protection of patients; and the performance of disease prevention and restorative measures. A RN is deemed competent in CAM therapies when she/he consistently demonstrates the knowledge of CAM therapies and performs these tasks safely.

The use of imagery as defined within the scope of nursing practice is a self-help educational model. It is the responsibility of the nurse not to only to stay within the scope of practice but within his or her practice competencies and expertise. If either of these conditions is not met, patients or clients should be referred to appropriate licensed health care professionals for imagery treatment. Techniques, such as the use of basic imagery scripts, relaxation, use of the breathing, and brief use of imagery (eg, "how would you imagine this antibiotic healing your infection," "if the pain could communicate with you, what would it say or want"), can be used by nurses without additional training; however, using the integrative imagery process should require education with a practicum that is supervised and meets specific competencies.

Use of imagery in nursing

The opportunities for use of imagery in nursing include every clinical setting in health care. Applications include but are not limited to control of pain, symptoms, and anxiety; preparation for labor, delivery, and surgery; augmenting the action of medication and treatment; minimizing side effects; dealing with chronic illness; optimizing healing; tolerating difficult procedures; accessing inner wisdom and guidance; accessing insights and information concerning a particular problem or situation; finding meaning in illness or crisis; accessing inner strengths; and coping with death and dying issues.

Imagery research and techniques

Guided imagery has been widely researched with positive effects over the past 25 years in many settings, but only two studies have been published with the use of integrative imagery. The two studies, one qualitative by Heinschel [13] and one quantitative by Scherwitz and colleagues [14], have paved the way for much needed replication in the interactive process between the imagery guide, patient, and image. The following use of techniques and citations of imagery research are some of the more frequently used applications in clinical settings.

Control of pain

There is virtually no arena in health care that is without the challenge of pain control. Any patient could be suffering from different experiences of pain, be it physical, emotional, social, or spiritual. Consider an elderly patient who has lost a limb to surgery, has no social support, must participate in physical therapy several times a day, and is grieving over the recent loss of a loved one. This scenario is not an unusual situation for the bedside nurse. A bolus of morphine may dull the physical pain, but there is always the chance of side effects and emotional suffering may still be present. Research has shown that the use of imagery techniques reduces the meaning of pain [15], increases self-efficacy for managing pain and improving functional status [16], and decreases the experience of pain and use of pain medications after surgery and invasive procedures [17–19].

Imagery approaches pain in several ways. The pain can be dealt with directly, modulated, altered, or used as an intervention to affect the pain. Some of the imagery techniques for pain control are exploring an image of the pain, imagining the pain and its relief, relaxation techniques, breathing methods, transforming pain using drawing and imagery, an intensity scale, accessing an inner strength or quality to help deal with the pain, altering the sensation or location of pain, and altering time before the pain was present or going to a future time when pain is relieved.

Control of anxiety

Anxiety and worry are frequent experiences for most of us. Upcoming surgery, a life-challenging diagnosis, change, loss, uncomfortable procedures, or the unknown of treatment outcomes greatly increases a patient's experience of anxiety. Imagery techniques have been shown to decrease anxiety about upcoming surgery [18], chemical dependency [20,21], difficult procedures and treatments [19], and coping with illness and pain [16]. In addition to many of the imagery techniques listed previously, the inner healer or inner wisdom technique represents an inner resource, protector, healer, ally, or higher power to an anxious patient.

Cancer care

The diagnosis of cancer often brings with it high levels of fear of death, uncertainty about recurrence, uncomfortable or unwanted treatments, and side effects of treatment. Patients often seek imagery because of these high levels of stress in the search for coping tools. Imagery research has demonstrated decreased anxiety, depression, and anticipatory nausea and vomiting before and after chemotherapy; improved quality of life [22,23]; and increased comfort during radiation therapy [24].

Once patients have achieved a sense of control by using imagery tools to cope and participate in their healing, they frequently have less anxiety and discomfort. Excellent resources for fighting cancer with imagery techniques are available in a book and compact disk (CD) by Rossman [25] and on CDs by Naparstek [26].

Cardiovascular disease and stroke

The immune system plays a role in the progression of coronary artery diseases and their clinical manifestations. It has been well established that chronic psychologic risk factors, such as hostility, low socioeconomic status, depression, exhaustion, mental stress, and anger, can promote myocardial ischemia and plaque rupture [27]. Imagery techniques, such as a peaceful place, and accessing inner strengths, such as patience and calmness, have been shown to decrease the effect of stressors. Clinical research has also demonstrated that imagery can reduce preoperative anxiety and postoperative pain among patients undergoing cardiac surgery [28].

Recent research is showing that imagery can play an important part in the rehabilitation of strokes and neurologic injury. Good outcomes have been found with relearning of daily tasks [29], the rehabilitation of hemiparesis, and motor tasks in general [30,31].

Imagery and pediatric care

Although the focus of this article is on adults, it should be mentioned that imagery does have may uses for children. In general, children are quick and eager to use imagery because it is much more a part of their daily life than with adults. The main difference is economy of words for the short attention span of children and the use of age-appropriate language. For example, pain control techniques translate into "ouch kits," in which the use of blowing bubbles can represent blowing pain out of the body or playing "puppies" helps a toddler in starting to ambulate as part of a game. Research supports significant decrease in pain and anxiety in children after surgery [32–34]. In addition, a book written by Curren [35], who is a nurse, tells the story of how imagery scripts that she and her daughter developed played a pivotal part in her child's healing.

Preparation for surgery

Preparing patients for surgery with scripted guided imagery audiotapes and CDs has been well used clinically and well researched over a long period. For the most part, the research outcomes have been quite positive. The most frequent results that have been replicated over time have demonstrated decreased anxiety and pain before and after surgery [36–41], less use of pain medications after surgery [18,19,34], fewer complications [18,19], increased wound healing [37,38,41], decreased length of stay [33,34,40,41], and decreased blood loss [38].

Imagery research, hospital programs, and individuals generally use prescripted guided imagery tapes and CDs. A hospital-based preparation for surgery program and the corresponding pilot study using integrative imagery are described elsewhere in this article.

Case examples

Nurses often raise the issue of not enough time to work with patients in clinical settings. It is true that there is a big difference in allotted time between an hour session in private practice and only 5 minutes on a busy nursing unit or clinic. The case examples described here demonstrate how effective and profound imagery can be, whether done briefly or in a full session. In addition, imagery gives the patients the tools they need and decreases burnout in the nurse. One of the major reasons why is that the nurse is not expending the energy of "fixing" the patient but rather teaching the patient self-care tools that the patient can then bring independently into his or her daily life.

Imagery in private practice

An actual case example exemplifies how imagery can not only alleviate physical pain but elicit an inner strength and give a client a self-care tool for life. A middle-aged woman who had been experiencing migraines since the recent loss of her husband came to the author's private practice. She stated that the migraines made her feel sick, helpless, lonely, and alone. She was first taught how to use her breath to initiate full-body relaxation. Her image for pain was a fist-sized pulsating ball of fire. When asked if she wanted to do anything with it, she said she was going to throw it into the ocean and then go to her favorite beach in Hawaii. Once at the beach, she felt the sun relax her entire body and listened to the sound of the waves. She was offered the technique of eliciting an inner strength that could help her to cope with her loneliness. She chose courage. After several days of rehearsing her "inner stage play" of breathing, relaxation, throwing the ball in the ocean, going to the beach, and feeling full of courage, she stopped having migraines. Seven years have passed, and there has been no reoccurrence of migraines.

Another case involved a young woman diagnosed with cancer of the esophagus. She learned many imagery tools over the 2 years of sessions that her friend paid for every 2 to 3 weeks. The following session not only gave the client the inner strength she needed to cope with her illness but became an unanticipated gift to the client and the practitioner much later. The client wanted to invite God into her special place of healing, her actual garden in her backyard. When God appeared in her imagery, she asked him to touch her and give her the inner strength she needed to cope with her many setbacks. Her pale face changed to a soft pink, and she smiled, with tears flowing down her face. Thereafter, the client used her inner garden to invite God to give her advice and support her in times of need. Two years later, her friend called to say that "Cathy" was in the hospital in a semicoma and probably would not last the night. The practitioner asked the friend to ask "Cathy" to go to her garden. The next morning, the friend called to say that "Cathy" had passed and said, "I told her to go to her garden and I saw a movement under the sheet and when I lifted the sheet, she was making an 'ok' sign with her fingers."

Brief imagery in clinical settings

An RN imagery guide enters a hospital room in which a patient is close to death. His large family is present, and his son is standing at the end of the bed holding a baby. The nurse asks the patient, "Is that baby your grandson?" The patient nods "yes." The nurse asks, "Does that little face bring you happiness?" The patient nods "yes." The nurse then asks "Would it bring you happiness to imagine this little face when you are alone or in any discomfort?" The patient nods "yes" and smiles. The family is smiling, along with some tears. End of session.

A patient is in an emergency room after sustaining a tension pneumothorax as well as a fractured leg and various other injuries. The patient is in extreme pain, and the RN imagery guide is asked to come in to help to restrain the patient for safety reasons. The physician was only able to give small amounts of pain medications because of the patient's shallow breathing. The nurse got close to the patient's head and had her imagine a place she wanted to be. The patient went to the beach and sat on the warm sand. The patient became quiet, and the other nurse, who was repositioning the leg, said, "Whatever you are doing up there, keep it up!" When the surgeon came in to insert a chest tube, the patient was offered a little more pain medication. The patient said to the nurse," I'm doing fine on the beach, I'm tuning out, just don't leave me."

A patient was scheduled to have an MRI scan and was expressing high anxiety because of claustrophobia An RN imagery guide asked the patient where he would rather be, and the patient responded, "in a duck blind hunting ducks." He was instructed on how to use all his senses in his mind's eye while having the test and to use the banging sound of the machine to keep him focused on the duck blind. The nurse was not able to accompany the patient to the radiology department, so he had to face the scanner alone with only the brief introduction to imagery. When the patient came back from the radiology department, the nurse asked how it went. He responded with a smile, "We're having duck for dinner."

Report of a successful hospital imagery program: a pilot study

In 2003, the Institute for Health and Healing (IHH) at Mills-Peninsula Health Services [42] hired the author and another holistic nurse who were certified in integrative imagery to provide imagery services to patients. A pilot study was designed to replicate the successful outcomes of the use of imagery in reducing pre- and postoperative anxiety and decreased use of pain medications after surgery. It was thought that with the visibility and credibility of the anticipated outcomes, there would be good support for offering imagery to all patients undergoing elective surgery.

The IHH medical director and the director of the Institutional Review Board at the hospital approved moving forward with the pilot program as a quality outcome study of patients undergoing elective knee and hip replacement. Twenty-nine patients received routine pre- and postoperative care, whereas 30 patients had an individualized preoperative imagery session, followed by listening to a scripted postoperative imagery audiotape. The imagery sessions were held 3 to 5 days before surgery. All the orthopedic patients were offered a free preoperative session. Those who asked for the imagery sessions were put in the intervention group, whereas those who were not interested were used as controls.

The patients in the intervention group received an imagery session after their preadmission appointment in the hospital. The patients were asked if they were experiencing any life stressors in their life or relevant to their upcoming surgery. Patients were told that the individualized imagery session would provide them with self-care tools that could reduce preoperative anxiety and stress and help them to manage postoperative pain in conjunction with pain medication. The control and intervention groups had patient controlled analgesia (PCA) devices per the usual orthopedic orders for this hospital. It was emphasized that not only would they learn and use these tools for the pre- and postoperative periods but that they would be able to apply them as self-care in their daily life.

The sessions included relaxation, a peaceful and calming place they had experienced or would like to experience, and rehearsal based on desired outcomes of surgery and imagery tools for any other challenges the patients identified. Once the words and images were obtained through some brief imagery, the session was recorded. The patients had an opportunity to debrief their experience and were then given the individualized audiotape to listen to before surgery and a generic tape for postoperative listening in the hospital and on into their recovery period after hospitalization. Patients were also visited on the day after surgery by the imagery nurses for follow-up as needed.

The pilot study was a replication of a study done by Tusek [18] and Lang and colleagues [19]. Outcome measures were pre- and postoperative levels of anxiety and pain and daily pain medication use after surgery. The traditional pain intensity scale was already in use at the hospital, with good documentation by the nursing staff. Nursing staff were also asked to document levels of anxiety using the same measurements as the pain scale; however, because of poor documentation, these had to be eliminated from the pilot results.

Results of the pilot study

The results of the study, as shown in Table 2, demonstrated a significant decrease in the perception of pain and daily use of opioid pain medication compared with the control group.

Telephone survey results

An imagery practitioner who was not involved in the pilot program volunteered to conduct a follow-up telephone survey. The summary of the survey results is shown in Table 3.

Table 2
Results of pilot research pain medication use in imagery subjects and controls

	N	Total opioid use administered intravenously (mg)	Average daily opioid use (mg)	Average perceived pain	Perceived pain after surgery	LOS
Imagery	29	90.20	18.80	3.10	2.00	4.76
Control	33	116.10	25.60	4.60	3.80	4.86
Significant results if $P < .05$	NA	0.089	0.049	0.001	0.000	0.304
		NS	Significant	Significant	Significant	NS

	Hips	Knees		Total
Control	18	15		33
Imagery	21	8		29

Abbreviations: LOS, level of significance; NS, not significant.
From Mills-Peninsula Health Services, Institute for Health and Healing, San Mateo, CA; with permission.

Table 3
Summary of telephone survey data

Questions	Yes	No
Did you receive any benefits from you imagery tape?	28	2
Decreased anxiety	14	
Decreased pain	12	
Relaxation	27	
Sleep	13	
Sense of control	6	
What did you like best about this program?		
Personal approach	26	
Tape session	16	
Individualized tape	12	
Postsurgery visits by imagery registered nurse	12	
What did you like least about this program?		
Tape quality	9	
Interruptions in hospital while listening to tape	10	
Needed more reminders to listen to tape	2	
Did you listen to your tape at home before surgery?	24	5
Did you listen to your tape everyday while in the hospital?	21	9
Are you still listening to your tape?	5	25
Would you recommend this program to someone else?	29	0
Would you write a letter of recommendation to administration?	20	9
May we quote you?	20	9

From Mills-Peninsula Health Services, Institute for Health and Healing, San Mateo, CA; with permission.

Postoperative patient comments

Additional comments from the telephone survey and from postoperative rounds are noted in Table 4.

Once the pilot study results were reported to the administrative, medical, and nursing staff of the hospital, all patients undergoing elective surgery were offered preoperative imagery sessions. Changes were made in the program based on the program evaluation from patients, such as a quiet office for the sessions; equipment to record CDs digitally; and staff reminders to encourage listening to the recordings when experiencing such stressors as anxiety, pain, and insomnia. The program continues to grow, with consistent high satisfaction ratings.

Additional hospital imagery services

Imagery is available to all inpatients and outpatients and to all hospital staff. Referrals mainly come from nursing staff, physicians, social workers, physical therapists, and hospital chaplains. The departments with the highest numbers of referrals are preadmission testing (for the preparation for surgery program), chemical dependency, acute rehabilitation, cancer center, orthopedics, and subacute nursing. There are beginning to be self-referring patients who have experienced imagery during a previous admission.

Table 4
Summary of patient comments on use of imagery

Strengths	Weaknesses
Put in right frame of mind	Tape had background noise (9)
Almost as effective as pain medications	Too drugged to listen to tape
Had headache in pre-admission testing (8/10); after tape (0/10)	Competing noises in hospital very distracting (15)
Helped me sleep	Hard to listen to tape uninterrupted (4)
Tape worked; helped me get away	Would have liked orthopedic nurses to remind me of tape (3)
Used tape after discharge to relax	
Tape helped me remember positive times	
Taped helped with hip pain and to sleep	
Like a vacation; the experience was wonderful	
I was more alert and did not require as much medication	
Quicker recovery	
Very innovative program	
Tape was a lifesaver	
Liked the personal visits by the imagery	
Nurses after surgery (5)	
Program was like a security blanket.	
Tape helped me to breathe properly when I was anxious	
I was able to be very relaxed and went home pain-free	
Put me in control; would have been terrified if not for the tape; my husband says, "they should have a drive-through at the hospital so all surgery patients can get a tape"	

From Mills-Peninsula Health Services, Institute for Health and Healing, San Mateo, CA; with permission.

Education for and imagery services are provided by the two part-time (one full-time equivalent) imagery nurses previously mentioned. Frequent imagery classes are also offered to the community, and continuing education unit classes are offered to hospital staff.

Costs

Inpatients are seen free of charge as a standard of care. Outpatients receive one free 1-hour session and pay a fee for service thereafter. Complementary therapies in hospitals and clinics continue to be at risk of being cut when budget constraints increase. At the present time, there has been no third party payment for imagery services. It is the strong feeling of the author and of the imagery patients and their families that an anxious, painful, exhausted, and upset patient is more expensive than a patient who feels that he or she has actively participated in his or her own healing.

Summary

Imagery is evidence based, can be used in all clinical settings, is safe, and gives the patient control over his or her internal environment. It is not a "fix-it" technique but rather a way of gifting patients with their own self-help tools. Once learned, it can be used the rest of a patient's life for management of stress, prevention, and well-being.

Imagery (indeed, all holistic practices) is underused in nursing. There is no order needed to initiate imagery, and its intervention has no side effects. Nursing is in a pivotal and respected pathway to model, teach, and pioneer holistic practice in the profession. Contributions in the area of imagery research, education, and implementation in the clinical setting are just a creative thought away.

References

[1] Reed T, Ezra S. Certificate program in integrative imagery handbook. Foster City (CA): Beyond Ordinary Nursing; 2003.

[2] Ader R, Felten D, Cohen S. Psychoneuroimmunology. New York: Academic Press; 1981.

[3] Fleshner M, Laudenslager M. Psychoneuroimmunology: then and now. Behav Cogn Neurosci Rev 2005;3(2):114–30.

[4] Starkweather A, Witek-Janusek L, Mathews H. Applying the psychoneuroimmunology framework to nursing research. J Neurosci Nurs 2005;37(1):56–62.

[5] McCain NL, Gray DP, Walter J, et al. Implementing a comprehensive approach to the study of health dynamics using the psychoneuroimmunology paradigm. ANS Adv Nurs Sci 2005; 28(4):320–32.

[6] McCain NL, Smith JC. Stress and coping in the context of psychoneuroimmunology: a holistic framework for nursing practice and research. Arch Psychiatr Nurs 1994;8(4):221–7.

[7] Bauer SM. Psychoneuroimmunology and cancer: an integrated review. J Adv Nurs 1994;19: 1114–20.

[8] Pert CB. Molecules of emotion. New York: Scribner; 1997.

[9] Rogers ME. Nursing: science of unitary irreducible human beings. In: Barrett EM, editor. Visions of Rogers' science-based nursing. New York: National League for Nursing; Update. 1990. p. 5–11.

[10] Beguslawsi M. Unitary human practice modalities. In: Barrett EM, editor. Visions of Rogers' science-based nursing. New York: National League for Nursing; Update. 1990. p. 83–92.

[11] American Holistic Nursing Association. Position on the role of nurses in the practice of complementary and alternative therapies. Available at: www.ahna.org/.

[12] California Board of Registered Nursing. Complementary and alternative therapies in registered nursing practice. 2000. Available at: www.rn.ca.gov. Accessed February 2000.

[13] Heinschel JA. A descriptive study of the interactive guided imagery experience. J Holist Nurs 2002;20:325–47.

[14] Scherwitz LW, McHenry P, Herrero R. Interactive guided imagery SM therapy with medical patients: predictors of health outcomes. J Altern Complement Med 2005;11(1):69–83.

[15] Lewandowski WA, Good M, Draucher CB. Changes in the meaning of pain with the use of guided imagery. Pain Manag Nurs 2005;6(2):58–67.

[16] Mezies V, Taylor A, Bourguenon C. Effects of guided imagery on outcomes of pain, functional states, and self-efficacy in persons diagnosed with fibromyalgia. J Altern Complement Med 2006;12(1):23–30.

[17] Lewandowski WA. Patterning of pain and power with guided imagery. Nurs Sci Q 2004; 17(3):233–41.

[18] Tusek D. Guided imagery: a significant advance in the care of patients undergoing elective colorectal surgery. Dis Colon Rectum 1997;40:172–8.

[19] Lang E, Benotsch E, Fick L, et al. Adjunctive non-pharmacological analgesia for invasive medical procedures: a randomized trial. Lancet 2000;355:1486–90.

[20] Kominars KD. A study of visualization and addiction treatment. J Subst Abuse Treat 1997; 14(3):213–23.

[21] Tusek D. Guided imagery: a powerful tool to decrease length of stay, anxiety, and narcotic consumption. J Invasive Cardiol 1999;11(4):265–7.

[22] Yoo HF, Ann SH, Kim SR, et al. Efficacy of progressive muscle relaxation training and guided imagery in reducing chemotherapy side effects in patients with breast cancer and in improving their quality of life. Support Care Cancer 2005;13(10):826–33.

[23] Raffel L, Schmidt K, Ernst E. A systematic review of guided imagery as an adjuvant cancer therapy. Psychooncology 2005;14(8):607–17.

[24] Kolcaba K, Fox C. The effects of guided imagery on comfort of women with early stage breast cancer undergoing radiation therapy. Oncol Nurs Forum 1999;26(1):67–72.

[25] Rossman ML. Fighting cancer from within. New York: Henry Holt & Co; 2003.

[26] Naparstek B. HealthJourneys: resources for mind, body and spirit. Available at: www.healthjourneys.com.

[27] Kop W. The integration of cardiovascular behavioral medicine and psychoneuroimmunology: new developments based on converging research fields. Brain Behav Immun 2003;17:233–7.

[28] Halpin LS, Speir AM, CapoBianco P, et al. Guided imagery in cardiac surgery. Outcomes Manag 2002;6(3):132–7.

[29] Lie KP, Lee RM, Chan CW. Mental imagery for promoting relearning for people after stroke: a randomized controlled trial. Arch Phys Med Rehabil 2004;85(9):1403–8.

[30] Stevens JA, Stay Kov MA. Using motor imagery in the rehabilitation of hemiparesis. Arch Phys Med Rehabil 2003;84(7):1090–2.

[31] Jackson PL, Lafleur MF, Malouin F, et al. Potential of mental practice using motor imagery in neurologic rehabilitation. Arch Phys Med Rehabil 2001;82(8):1133–41.

[32] Huth MM, Broome ME, Good M. Imagery reduces children's post-operative pains. Pain 2004;110(1–2):439–48.

[33] Ball TM, Shapiro DE, Monheim CJ, et al. A pilot study of the use of guided imagery for the treatment of recurrent abdominal pain in children. Clin Pediatr (Phila) 2003;42(6):527–32.

[34] Lambert SA. The effects of hypnosis/guided imagery on the postoperative course of children. J Dev Behav Pediatr 1996;17(5):307–10.

[35] Curren E. Guided imagery for healing children and teens. Oregon (OR): Beyond Words Publishing; 2001.

[36] Tusek D, Church JM, Fazio VW. Guided imagery as a coping strategy for perioperative patients. AORN J 1997;66(4):644–9.

[37] Holden-Lund C. Effects of radiation with guided imagery on surgical stress and wound healing. Res Nurs Health 1988;11:235–44.

[38] Dreher H. Mind-body interventions for surgery: evidence and exigency. Adv Mind Body Med 1998;14:207–22.

[39] Laurion S, Fetzer SJ. The effect of two nursing interventions on the postoperative outcomes of gynecologic laparoscopic patients. J Perianesth Nurs 2003;18(4):254–61.

[40] Antall GF, Kresevic D. The use of guided imagery to manage pain in an elderly orthopaedic population. Orthop Nurs 2004;23(5):335–40.

[41] Miller T. The value of perioperative nursing. Semin Perioper Nurs 1998;7(2):108–13.

[42] Mills-Peninsula Health Service, Institute for Health and Healing. San Mateo (CA). Available at: www.mills-peninsula.org.

ELSEVIER
SAUNDERS

NURSING
CLINICS
OF NORTH AMERICA

Nurs Clin N Am 42 (2007) 279–293

Meeting Clients' Spiritual Needs

Cheryl Delgado, PhD, RN, ANP-BC

*School of Nursing, Cleveland State University, 2121 Euclid Avenue,
RT 910, Cleveland, OH 44115, USA*

It is commonly accepted that nursing approaches health care from a holistic point of view as opposed to a reductionist model. Descartian dualism, artificially separating body and mind/spirit, is not compatible with understanding the person as a whole integrated being in continuing interaction with internal and external environments. Yet, although much progress has been made in learning about a person's physical functions and needs, nursing and other sciences have found the cognitive, emotional, and spiritual aspects of being more difficult to explore. Because it is so intertwined with all other aspects of the person, we may have difficulty in finding a perspective that reveals more than a fragment of the person's spirituality at a time, and because we each have our own spiritual point of view, each of us sees through a unique lens of understanding. This article has four main purposes. It offers some insight into the historical perspective and the meaning and importance of spirituality for nursing, briefly reviews current literature focusing on spiritual care and spiritual needs assessments, identifies barriers to providing spiritual care, and summarizes spiritual care interventions that have been effectively used to meet patients' needs. It is intended to be the start of an open exchange of ideas rather than the final word on the subject.

Historical perspective and importance of spirituality to nursing

Caring for the spiritual needs of a person must be at least as old as and may predate caring for the physical needs. Those who led families or groups of early peoples were men and women believed to have special understanding and the power to restore spiritual harmony or balance. Ancient texts in Egypt refer to priest physicians, old Chinese writings mention lay attendants for the sick who functioned as nurses [1], and there are biblical references to nurses and midwives (eg, Genesis 24:59, Exodus 1:15). Although there were

E-mail address: c.delgado@csuohio.edu

few effective curative therapies, there is evidence of ritual practices concerned with creating, maintaining, and transcending life [2]. Fertility offerings; amulets to ward off illness; and cleansing rites at puberty, childbirth, and death demonstrate that healing was then, as now, holistic.

The Saxon root word *halean* or *hal*, meaning whole, is the source of the English words heal, health, whole, and holy and is related to the Greek *holos*, meaning entire or whole. Burkhardt [3] notes that healing is a process beyond curing because it is grounded in equal consideration of the physical, emotional, and spiritual concerns, and Glueck [4] debated whether one could be healthy without being spiritually whole or "holy."

The definition of health by the World Health Organization states that health is a state of complete well-being physically, mentally, and socially and is not limited to a disease-free condition. This definition subsumes spiritual care within the mandate for mental and social wellness. Nursing has the responsibility to understand the human responses to illness and to engage in activities that are preventative as well as restorative in all three of the World Health Organization's areas of concern.

Some nursing theories have explicit statements about meeting spiritual needs (eg, those of Nightingale, Neuman, Leininger, Roy, and Watson), whereas other theories speak indirectly to the matter (eg, those of Parse and Newman). Theories from disciplines other than nursing also support the importance of providing spiritual care. Frankl [5] has influenced nurses studying persons with serious illness, life meanings, and positive attitudes, and nurses have used the stress and coping frameworks of Antonovsky, Lazarus, and Folkman to research spiritual responses to illness [6,7].

Professional organizations give support for spiritual care. The North American Nursing Diagnosis Association (NANDA) recognizes a nursing diagnosis of spiritual distress and suggests nursing interventions classification (NIC) [8]. The American Nurses Association's code of ethics for nurses [9] requires that nurses consider the person's value system and religious beliefs in planning and providing health care, and the International Council of Nurses' code for nurses [10] also specifically mentions spiritual beliefs. The Joint Commission on Accreditation for Healthcare Organizations (JCAHO) specifies that all patients be assessed for spiritual beliefs and have spiritual support available [11]. The American Association of Colleges of Nursing recommends that nursing education prepare nurses to comprehend the meaning of spirituality in relation to health and healing [12]. Responding to spiritual needs would clearly seem to be an expectation in practice, yet nursing texts contain only a few scattered references to spiritual care [13,14].

The nursing diagnosis of spiritual distress is noted to be related to anxiety and stress, losses and suffering, and separation from or challenges to a belief system. Evidence of spiritual distress may be seen as concern with death, inner conflict about belief systems (sometimes expressed as anger oriented toward a deity, self-blame, or nonparticipation in one's usual spiritual activities), somatic complaints, or active requests for spiritual assistance [15]. In crisis, patients and families may attempt to find meaning in suffering or assign causality for their illness. This period may result in loss of faith or may result in spiritual growth, and the nurse's response to the patient can be vital [16].

Identifying spiritual needs

In interviews with elderly patients in a geriatric ward in Scotland, six men and four women described their spiritual needs. They were concerned with religious needs (eg, prayer, reading the Bible, attending church), finding sense and meaning in life, sharing love and belonging, and the need for moral standing (eg, treating people well, doing the right thing) and had questions about life after death [17].

Hermann's [18] qualitative study of elderly patients with cancer who were terminally ill described 29 different spiritual needs falling into six themes. They were religious practices, companionship, involvement and control, experiencing nature, having a positive outlook, and finishing business. Completing unfinished business and discussing the difference between grief and guilt, helping the patient to deal with and find forgiveness of self, are significant nursing interventions [15,19]. Cavendish and colleagues [20] reported that determining meaning in past experiences and current situations through reflection and being open to patients' feelings about illness and death were nursing activities used by Sigma Theta Tau members.

There seems to be agreement in the literature that a definition of spiritual needs commonly identifies three basic or fundamental concerns: the need to find meaning in illness or disability; the need to affirm one's relationship or connect with others (including nature or a Supreme Other); and the need to realize transcendent values, such as hope, faith, trust, courage, love, and peace [21]. It should be noted that these needs, although spiritual, are not necessarily religious.

There is a danger in the current focus of spirituality in the West on Judeo-Christian values. Our diverse society is multicultural, multiracial, and multireligious. Nurses care for patients with many different, and sometimes no, faith systems. Henley and Schott [22] identified spiritual universals across several belief traditions and humanism. It is generally agreed that persons have a soul or spirit (a spiritual dimension), that life is sacred, and that life has a higher purpose. Fundamental shared values include doing what is right, including being truthful and fulfilling family duties. Prayer, meditation, or other reflective acts are common practices.

There is often confusion about spirituality and religion. There is a strong connection between the two and a significant difference. A mature religiosity may enhance spirituality, and many persons find expression of their spirituality through religious activities, but others find expression through nontheologic humanistic beliefs [23]. Spirituality comprises a wide range of metaphysic beliefs and is broader in scope than religion, which relies on a formalized belief system manifested through ritual behaviors. Spirituality is inclusive in nature, embracing connection with others, including a deity if that is within the belief system. Religion may be elitist and exclusive in nature, as in the "true" way, the "chosen," or the "One." Faith, as an acknowledgment of unseen power, is evident in both, but there is a danger that rigidity and uncompromising dogma may create anxiety and fear rather than provide comfort and succor. Patients who perceive that they are unable to satisfy religious requirements may experience increased stress rather than comfort from their beliefs.

Spiritual assessments

Before spiritual needs can be met, spiritual needs must be recognized. Initially, assessing spiritual needs consisted of documenting the patient's religious affiliation, but Stoll [24] and Highfield [25] expanded the assessment to include exploration of preferred religious practices, the patient's beliefs on sources of hope and strength, and the relation of the patient's spirituality to health. Since 1990, 21 articles giving advice on spiritual assessment have been published in core nursing journals, and other disciplines, such as medicine, psychiatry, psychology and pastoral care, have added suggestions. Few of these have actually been tested.

In 2002, McSherry and Ross [26] published a literature review of spiritual assessment tools, finding variations ranging from descriptive accounts to in-depth spiritual histories. They noted that instruments were commonly used in initial assessments but suggested that continuous ongoing assessments made by nurses who have established rapport and trust with a patient using open-ended questions may most accurately reveal an individual's spiritual needs.

Questionnaires often contain multiple items and may be difficult to understand and tiring to complete. Of nine published spiritual assessment tools reviewed for this writing, two contain more than 50 items [24,27], five contain 20 to 30 items [28,29], and one suggests open-ended questions in four major areas [28]. Lengthy assessments could be problematic in initial contacts with acutely ill patients and in other circumstances in which time is a concern or when the patient's physical condition is fragile. Direct in-depth questions on matters of spirituality or religion may be viewed as intrusive [26] or totally inappropriate in situations in which the focus must be on prompt implementation of life-saving measures.

A consideration in using an assessment tool is the degree to which the instrument focuses on religious beliefs. Catteral and colleagues [30] and Johnson [31] agree that assessments must be appropriate for all persons, irrespective of religious affiliation, and for persons who profess no religious beliefs. Some instruments report lower scores for persons without a religious affiliation [32], indicating that the measure may address religion rather than spirituality.

Regardless of whether spiritual assessment is done as part of the admission process or in response to the nurse's awareness that the patient is exhibiting evidence of spiritual distress, the nurse may initiate assessment with a simple open-ended question. This indicates the nurse's willingness to assist the patient and allows the patient to articulate his or her concerns. Some patients do not broach the subject of spirituality with nonpastoral health care providers because they believe nurses and physicians are more concerned with physical care. In a study of spiritual coping mechanisms in 15 chronically ill men and women in the United Kingdom, some felt that they had to conceal spiritual beliefs and practices to avoid becoming an object of ridicule about them [33]. This may be even more of a problem when the patient's religious or spiritual beliefs are different from those of the mainstream community.

Challenges in providing spiritual care

Narayanasamy [34] wrote more than a decade ago that nurses were aware of patients' spiritual needs but poorly met them and suggested more education in spiritual care. In a study of oncology, among parish and hospice nurses, only 15% had learned spiritual care in nursing education [35]. Other researchers have described nurses as involved in providing spiritual care but not as leaders [36,37]. Nurses have expressed confidence in their ability to provide physical care but lack confidence in providing spiritual care [38,39]. The nurse's personal spirituality and knowledge to support spiritual care were found to be important factors for hospice nurses in confidence and competence in spiritual caregiving [40].

Other barriers to providing spiritual care have been identified. McEwen [41] broadly classed barriers into three categories: personal, situational, and knowledge related. Some nurses were uncomfortable with or uncertain of their own spirituality or saw spiritual needs as a private or pastoral responsibility. Some felt there was insufficient time because of the press of other care duties or restrictions from employers. Additionally, the immediate environment of the patient was not always conducive to addressing personal or spiritual concerns.

McEwen [41] also found that some nurses felt unable to differentiate psychologic needs from spiritual needs and had received little information during their nursing education on spiritual and religious matters. Similar concerns and other difficulties were uncovered in a study by Vance [42] on nurses' attitudes toward spirituality and patient care. Some nurses perceived a barrier to providing for spiritual needs if the nurse and patient did not share a common belief system, perhaps related to issues of evangelism or proselytizing and the concern that some interventions might be interpreted as unprofessional. Prayer with patients can be controversial. Emblen and Pesut [43] recommend that prayer with patients is appropriate when initiated by the patient but possibly coercive when initiated by the nurse.

Although often mentioned as a nursing intervention, prayer has been found to be one of the least preferred interventions by patients [44].

There is evidence that patients do not recognize spiritual care as a nursing activity. Davis [45] found that nine of the eleven persons interviewed in her phenomenologic study of patient expectations did not expect spiritual care from nurses and that one was adamantly opposed to it. Patients expected that the extent of the nurse's involvement was to call a chaplain, and although they noted activities indicative of presence (eg, touching, exhibiting concern and caring, listening, sharing self), these were interpreted as good nursing care and not spiritual care. Taylor and Mamier [46] surveyed 156 patients with cancer and 68 of their caregivers, mostly Christian, finding that they had widely varying expectations of spiritual care, with a preference for interventions that were less intimate, nonreligious in nature, and commonly used.

Meeting spiritual needs: review of the literature

Recently, there has been an increase in the amount of research devoted to meeting spiritual care needs. Publications in the 1990s identified nursing interventions to meet spiritual needs that can be placed in three major classifications. The most frequently mentioned interventions were aimed at communication with or aiding in the process of connecting to others or a Supreme Other, such as listening, building trust, touch, and being present. The second most often cited interventions were activities that facilitated religious or spiritual activities, such as prayer, meditation, and arranging for ritual needs (eg, administration of sacraments, accommodation of dietary restrictions). Referral, through arranging for a pastoral visit or informing the patient of other available resources, was also a common type of intervention.

In a survey of 176 American nurses, Piles [39] found that the provision of spiritual care was related to several factors. Nurses who felt confident in their ability to provide spiritual care did so more often than other nurses and had exposure to spiritual care in their nursing education. The nurse's perception of obstacles to providing care and the difficulty of separating psychologic and spiritual concerns also affected the nurse's likelihood of engaging in spiritual care, although more than 95% felt that holistic care included addressing spiritual concerns. No interventions were tested, but discussion of spiritual matters, prayer and scripture reading, and referral to clergy were suggested.

Clarke and colleagues [47], in a qualitative study of 15 persons after hospitalization, found three interventions directly involving patients and two directed toward policies and spiritual care. The direct measures were establishing a trusting relationship, providing a supportive environment, and responding sensitively to patients' beliefs. The policy actions were to integrate spirituality into the quality assurance plan and to emphasize the nurse's key role in the health care system.

In a comparison of spiritual needs and interventions by patients, nurses, and clergy, five nursing actions were recognized: prayer, scripture, presence, listening, and referral [48]. Oncology nurses, hospice nurses, and parish nurses used these interventions but also identified conveying acceptance and instilling hope as important [39]. Taylor and colleagues' [49] quantitative descriptive study of oncology nurses and spiritual care practices added depth by the inclusion of the family as therapeutically significant.

Since the millennium, the amount of published research on spiritual care has dramatically increased. The three most frequently cited nursing interventions in the literature after 2000 indicate a subtle but important shift. A review of the literature reveals that communicating effectively with and facilitating the patient to connect with others through such actions as active listening, presence, actively exploring the patient's spirituality, comforting with words and physical contact, reminiscing, supporting, and demonstrating respect were the most frequently used interventions. This indicates that excellent therapeutic communication skills are currently the primary intervention for meeting patients' spiritual needs.

Assisting the patient to engage in religious or other spiritual activities remained the second most frequently used nursing activity. Referring to clergy; informing patients of resources; providing religious materials; allowing for prayer, meditation, or music; and helping the patient to attend religious services are activities in this category.

The third category is concerned with the provision of physical care. Perhaps influenced by the recognition that physical contact, such as touch, can be therapeutic, nurses are increasingly aware that providing exemplary care for the patient's physical needs and relieving pain allow the patient to replace negative feelings with a more positive attitude. In a study of nearly 300 bedside nurses at a university hospital, Grant [50] found that almost all nurses believed that spirituality could give their patients "inner peace, strength to cope, bring about physical relaxation and self awareness, and help them forgive, connect and cooperate with others ... reduce bodily pain ... (and) facilitate physical healing."

Studies of chronically ill persons find that with advancing age or terminal illness, persons increase their focus on spiritual or religious concerns [51,52]. One study found that nurses themselves are more sensitive to spiritual needs when patients are elderly or terminally ill [53]. Grieving over loss (actual and potential), adjusting to altered roles, dealing with disabilities, and recognizing one's own mortality have been identified as coping tasks of chronically ill adults by Miller [54], who also noted that chronically ill persons needed respite from suffering and feelings of isolation, stating that "Spiritual malaise does not appear to be conducive to healing." Recent research validates that perception. In a study of long-term cancer survivors, Killoran and colleagues [55] found that all acknowledged a sense of spirituality and personal determination. Dewar and Lee [56] and Sowell and colleagues [7] found spirituality to be a significant resource for coping in devastating illnesses.

Spiritual nursing actions involve relieving patients' emotional distress. Vassalo [57] noted that nurses caring for patients dying at home used caring rather than curing behaviors. Relieving the patient's fears and feelings of vulnerability by explaining the medical plan of care can be supportive of spiritual well-being [45]. Acknowledging the patient's concerns, putting matters into perspective, clarifying meaning, and displaying nonjudgmental empathy are all supportive interventions [58,59].

The model for spiritual care proposed by Emblen and Pesut [43] suggests the careful use of humor as a strategy to promote emotional comfort. More than 80% of nurses responding to one survey had used laughter to provide support [50]. Patients in one study noted that helping them to laugh or sharing humor was a positive spiritual nursing intervention [46]. Using humor to establish a relationship and to relieve anger and tension can be effective if thoughtfully done [20].

Humor was not a strategy used by the 52 nurses surveyed by Narayanasamy and colleagues [19]. Interventions identified in this study were using personal religious beliefs to help patients, observation of religious beliefs and practices, respect for privacy, helping patients to connect, helping patients to complete unfinished business, listening to patients' concerns, and comforting and reassuring.

Several other studies emphasized the importance of creating a climate that communicated respect, aiding the patient in maintaining meaningful relationships and providing a circle of support (connectedness) [38,60]. Providing spiritual care has been seen as a way of using simple human ways to understand meaning and purpose in life [38], and several reflections on spiritual care have opined that the quality of the relationship between the patient and nurse is pivotal in providing spiritual care [61–63]. Sellers' [64] qualitative ethnographic study points out that nurses can enhance spirituality by understanding the unique human experience of each patient through a caring nurse-patient relationship characterized by the art of being present, respecting, and giving of self.

Van Leeuwen and Cusveller [58] have developed a competency profile for nurses in The Netherlands. They used a qualitative literature review to outline three domains (awareness of self, nursing process, and quality of expertise) and six core competencies (understanding one's personal beliefs, addressing the subject, information collection, discussion and planning, provision and evaluation of care, and integration into policy). Their conclusions emphasize the need for education on spiritual care issues and the need for multidisciplinary cooperation.

Implications for care

In summary, the extant literature on meeting spiritual needs identifies three broad classifications of nursing actions: assessment, communication, and support. Fig. 1 provides a model for spiritual care in which the person

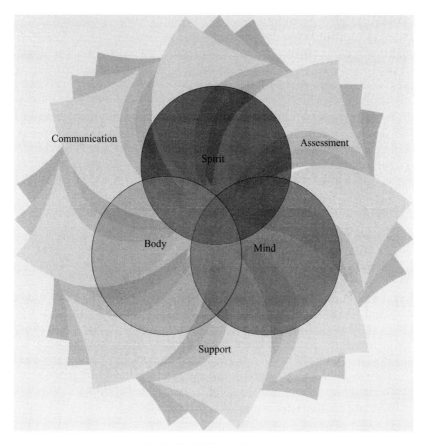

Fig. 1. Model for spiritual care.

is embraced within a spiritual environment. The nonlinear character of spiritual care is represented as an intertwined braid of assessment, communication, and support. Box 1 provides examples of specific interventions suggested from the literature review in each of these broad areas.

The assessment of spiritual needs requires nurses initially to understand their own spiritual condition. Acknowledging this, they must next be willing to bracket personal beliefs and direct attention to the patient. Using assessment tools or open-ended questions, the faith system, practices, and symbolic meanings of the patient need to be identified. Open-ended questions useful in a spiritual assessment include the following:

Do you think of yourself as a spiritual or religious person?
Tell me about spiritual or religious beliefs that are important to you.
Does the present situation (or illness) interfere with spiritual or religious activities that are important to you?
What spiritual or religious practices do you find most comforting?

Box 1. Spiritual interventions

Assessment
    Asking questions about faith, practices, and symbols
    Probing meanings for the patient
    Using assessment tools, questionnaires, and interviewing[a]
    Distinguishing spiritual needs/problems from pathologic
       conditions
Communication
    Listening[a]
    Clarifying meaning
    Focusing on the patient's spirituality or world view
    Informing the patient about spiritual resources (eg, clergy,
       availability for conversations, services)[a]
    Communicating patient's needs to other professionals
    Creating continuity of care
    Communicating with/involving family and friends
    Showing acceptance and respect for the patient's beliefs
    Self knowledge of nurse's own beliefs
    Avoiding evangelism
Supporting
    Emotionally
        Watching over the patient after bad news
        Putting things into perspective
        Not giving false hope
        Comforting emotional suffering
        Presence
        Trust
        Empathy
        Calmness
        Unselfish attention
        Referring to other professionals
    Physically
        Creating conditions (eg, time room, resources)
          for spiritual needs, activities, and rituals[a]
        Being near, present, touch
        Giving competent physical care
        Alleviating physical suffering

---

[a] Indicates intervention from NANDA NIC.

Is there anyone you would like to see or talk to? May I assist in arranging a visit?

Can you share your feelings with me?

What can I do to help you at this time?

Differentiation between spiritual needs and psychologic pathologic conditions should be made during this process.

Therapeutic communication skills are important in the assessment and subsequent interactions for spiritual care. Focusing on the patient's spirituality and the avoidance of evangelism demonstrate acceptance and respect for the patient's beliefs. Active listening and focused presence mean paying attention to the words that are spoken and the words that are not. Authenticity means that the nurse is engaged with the person and not merely performing the task of data collection. Effective communication builds trust and a strong patient-nurse relationship. Effective communication also fosters connection.

It is axiomatic that in a holistic framework, all things are connected. Ornish [65] proposes that anything leading to separation, isolation, and alienation contributes to illness and suffering and that which promotes intimacy and connection is healing. Spirituality involves communion within the self, with others, with nature, and with a Transcendent Other (if that is within the patient's beliefs).

Nurses may find that touch, a physical contact with the patient that expresses caring, fosters connection. Historically, healing traditions have used touch or the laying on of hands as a diagnostic and therapeutic process, and Burkhardt and Nagai-Jacobson [27] consider touch essential for the overall development of well-being. Nurses use touch in varied ways ranging from simply holding a distressed patient's hand to energy-based massage therapies.

Connecting with the transcendent is more difficult because it requires stepping beyond the physical. The common religious practices of prayer and meditation are essentially reflective cognitive processes and a fundamental way to connect with one's inner self and with a Transcendent Other. Prayer and meditation characteristically lead to physical relaxation and an opening of the consciousness beyond the here and now. Studies have shown that physical changes associated with prayer and meditation promote health and reduce stress [66,67]. Prayer, like meditation, is perceived by many as a private action, and although many patients are not comfortable praying with a health care provider, some are open to being prayed for. Learning the prayer preferences of the patient is part of the spiritual needs assessment.

Communicating the patient's or family's needs with others is a communication that aids communion or connecting. Involving family and friends as appropriate and informing the patient about spiritual care resources, such as the availability of clergy or the opportunity to participate in services, are ways to demonstrate respect for the patient's beliefs and promote continuity and stability in the patient's spiritual life. Spiritual needs are more often exacerbated than diminished by illness, and isolation of the patient from comforting spiritual practices can occur with confinement in an institutional setting or even if the patient becomes housebound.

Creating conditions that promote connection to a faith community and participation in valued spiritual practices can augment other supportive nursing actions. Supportive spiritual nursing interventions may be physical or emotional. Touching and providing competent physical care are physical expressions of support. Maintaining a relationship of trust and empathy, providing calm, honestly answering concerns without giving false hope, putting things into perspective, and watching over a patient in distress are nurturing emotional interventions.

Presence has been described as a spiritual intervention [48,49,63,68], but it is not often explained. Burkhardt and Nagai-Jacobson [27] describe presence as "a way of being physically, emotionally, and energetically with another in a way that conveys our willingness to hear, to know, to appreciate, and to receive who the other is and what the person is experiencing in this moment." It is sharing authentic awareness of the other and a nonjudgmental attention to the true nature of the other. Being in true presence with another is a unique connection of the spirits.

Nurses are, by the nature of their almost continual contact with patients and the intimacy of the patient-nurse relationship, well positioned to assess the spiritual concerns of their patients and have a wide range of spiritual interventions to use in meeting spiritual needs. Nurses recognize that holistic care includes meeting spiritual needs but may feel ill-prepared to address these concerns with patients or may feel that to offer support may be construed as promoting their own personal beliefs. As a profession, nursing needs to foster research in discovering optimal strategies for spiritual support and to educate all nurses to provide for spiritual needs.

Curing and *healing* are terms that may be used interchangeably in modern health care, but healing and curing are not the same. Curing is to be rid of or correct a disease process, but not all conditions can be cured. All persons can experience healing. Self-awareness, personal growth, and transcendence of bodily concerns characterize healing, even though pathologic conditions may remain. Healing needs and spiritual needs are often one and the same. If spiritual concerns are neglected, the healing process cannot move forward.

References

[1] Ackerknecht EH. A short history of medicine. Baltimore (MD): The Johns Hopkins University Press; 1982.
[2] Torrance RM. The spiritual quest: transcendence and myth, religion and science. Berkeley (CA): University of California Press; 1994. p. 61–8.
[3] Burkhardt MA. Spirituality: an analysis of the concept. Holist Nurs Pract 1989;3(3):69–77.
[4] Glueck N. Religion and health: a theological discussion. J Relig Health 1988;27(2):109–18.

[5] Frankl V. Man's search for meaning. New York: Washington Square Press; 1985.

[6] Coward D. Self transcendence and correlates in a healthy population. Nurs Res 1996;45(2): 116–21.

[7] Sowell R, Moneyham L, Guillory J, et al. Spiritual activities as a resistance resource for women with human immunodeficiency virus. Nurs Res 2000;49(2):73–81.

[8] North American Nursing Diagnosis Association. NANDA diagnosis: definitions and classification; spiritual distress 2005–6. Philadelphia: NANDA International.

[9] Code of ethics for nurses with interpretive statements. Washington, DC: American Nurses Association. 2001. p. 7.

[10] International Council of Nurses code of ethics for nurses. Geneva (Switzerland): International Council of Nurses; 2006.

[11] Available at: http://www.jointcommission.org/AccreditationPrograms/Hospitals/Standards/ FAQs. Accessed September 28, 2006.

[12] Essentials of college and university education for professional nursing. Washington, DC: American Association of Colleges of Colleges of Nursing; 1986.

[13] Smeltzer SC, Bare BG. Brunner and Suddarth's textbook of medical surgical nursing. 9th edition. Philadelphia: Lippincott; 2000.

[14] Ignatavicius DD, Workman ML. Medical surgical nursing: critical thinking for collaborative care. Philadelphia: W.B. Saunders Company; 2002.

[15] Doenges ME, Moorhouse MF, Geissler-Murr AC. Nursing care plans. Philadelphia: FA Davis; 2000. p. 350.

[16] Byrne M. Spirituality in palliative care: what language do we need? Int J Palliat Nurs 2002; 8(2):67–74.

[17] Ross LA. Elderly patients' perceptions of their spiritual needs and care: a pilot study. J Adv Nurs 1993;26:710–5.

[18] Hermann CP. Spiritual needs of dying patients: a qualitative study. Oncol Nurs Forum 2001; 28(1):67–72.

[19] Narayanasamy A, Clissert P, Parumal L, et al. Responses to spiritual needs of older people. J Adv Nurs 2004;48(1):6–16.

[20] Cavendish B, Konecny L, Mitzeloitis C, et al. Spiritual care activities of nurses using nursing interventions classifications (NIC) labels. Int J Nurs Terminol Classif 2003;14(4):113–24.

[21] Wright LM. Spirituality, suffering and illness: ideas for healing. Philadelphia: FA Davis Co; 2005.

[22] Henley A, Schott J. Culture, religion and patient care in a multiethnic society. London: Age Concern; 1999.

[23] Delgado C. A discussion of the concept of spirituality. Nurs Sci Q 2005;18(2):157–62.

[24] Stoll RI. Guidelines for spiritual assessment. Am J Nurs 1979;79:1574–7.

[25] Highfield MF, Cason C. Spiritual needs of patients: are they recognized? Cancer Nurs 1983; 6(3):187–92.

[26] McSherry W, Ross L. Dilemmas of spiritual assessment: considerations for nursing practice. J Adv Nurs 2002;38(5):479–88.

[27] Burkhardt MA, Nagai-Jacobson MG. Healing and spirituality. In: Spirituality: living our connectedness. Albany (NY): Delmar; 2002. p. 25–9.

[28] Taylor EJ. Spiritual care: nursing theory, research and practice. Upper Saddle River (NJ): Prentice Hall; 2002.

[29] Piedmont R. Does spirituality represent the sixth factor of personality? Spiritual transcendence and the five factor model. J Pers 1999;67(6):985–1013.

[30] Catteral RA, Cox M, Greet B, et al. The assessment and audit of spiritual care. Int J Palliat Nurs 1998;4(4):162–8.

[31] Johnson CP. Assessment tools: are they an effective approach to implementing spiritual health care within the NHS? Accid Emerg Nurs 2001;9:177–86.

[32] Reed PG. Religiousness among terminally ill and healthy adults. Res Nurs Health 1986;9: 35–41.

[33] Narayanasamy A. Spiritual coping mechanisms in chronic illness: a qualitative study. J Clin Nurs 2004;13:116–7.

[34] Narayanasamy A. Nurses' awareness and educational preparation in meeting the patient's spiritual needs. Nurse Educ Today 1993;13(3):196–201.

[35] Sellers SC, Haag BA. Spiritual nursing interventions. Journal of Holistic Care 1998;16(3): 338–54.

[36] Highfield MF. PLAN: a spiritual care model for every nurse. Quality of Life 1993;2(3):80–4.

[37] Babler JE. A comparison of spiritual care provided by hospice social workers, nurses and spiritual care professionals. Hosp J 1997;12(4):15–27.

[38] Meyerhoff H, VanHofwegen L, Harwood CH, et al. Emotional rescue: spiritual nursing interventions. Can Nurse 2002;98(3):21.

[39] Piles CL. Providing spiritual care. Nurse Educ 1987;15(1):36–41.

[40] Belcher A, Griffiths M. The spiritual care perspectives and practices of hospice nurses. Journal of Hospice and Palliative Nursing 2005;7(5):271–9.

[41] McEwen M. Spiritual nursing care: state of the art. Holist Nurs Pract 2005;19(4):161–8.

[42] Vance DL. Nurses' attitudes toward spirituality and patient care. Medsurg Nurs 2001;10(5): 264–8.

[43] Emblen J, Pesut B. Strengthening transcendent meaning: a model for the spiritual nursing care of patients experiencing suffering. J Holist Nurs 2001;19(1):42–56.

[44] Bauer T, Barron CR. Nursing interventions for spiritual care: preferences of the community based elderly. J Holist Nurs 1995;13(3):268–79.

[45] Davis LA. A phenomenological study of patient expectations concerning nursing care. Holist Nurs Pract 2005;19(3):126–33.

[46] Taylor E, Mamier I. Spiritual care nursing: what cancer patients and family caregivers want. J Adv Nurs 2005;49(3):260–7.

[47] Clarke C, Cross J, Deane, et al. Spirituality: integral to quality care. Holist Nurs Pract 1991; 5(3):67–76.

[48] Emblen JD, Halstead L. Spiritual needs and interventions: comparing the views of patients, nurses and chaplains. Clin Nurse Spec 1993;7(4):175–83.

[49] Taylor EJ, Amenta M, Highfield MF. Spiritual care practices of oncology nurses. Oncol Nurs Forum 1995;22:31–9.

[50] Grant D. Spiritual interventions: how when and why nurses use them. Holist Nurs Pract 2004;18(1):36–41.

[51] Courtenay BC, Poon LW, Martin P, et al. Religiosity and adaptation in the oldest-old. Int J Aging Hum Dev 1992;34(1):47–56.

[52] Bowes DE, Tamlyn D, Butler LJ. Women living with ovarian cancer: dealing with an early death. Health Care Women Int 2001;23:135–48.

[53] Dettmore DF. Nurses' conceptions of and practices in the spiritual dimension of nursing [doctoral dissertation]. Columbia University Teachers College; Dissertation Abstracts International; 1986. p. 47.

[54] Miller JF. Coping with chronic illness: overcoming powerlessness. Philadelphia: FA Davis Co; 2000.

[55] Killoran M, Schlitz MJ, Lewis NR. Unremarkable recoveries: normalizing adversary and cancer survival. Qualitative Health Research 2002;12(2):208–22.

[56] Dewar AL, Lee EA. Bearing illness and injury. West J Nurs Res 2000;22(8):912–28.

[57] Vassalo BM. The spiritual aspects of dying at home. Holist Nurs Pract; 15(2): 17–29.

[58] Van Leeuwen R, Cusveller B. Nursing competencies for spiritual care. J Adv Nurs 2004; 48(3):234–46.

[59] Tanyi RA. Spirituality and family nursing: spiritual assessment and interventions for families. J Adv Nurs 2006;53(3):287–94.

[60] Treolar LL. Integration of spirituality into health care practice by nurse practitioners. J Am Acad Nurse Pract 2000;12(7):280–5.

[61] Page M. How well do we care for people's spiritual needs. Kai Tiaki Nuring 2005;Nov:18–9.

[62] Hudson R, Rumbold B. Spiritual care. In: O'Connor M, Aranda S, editors. Palliative nursing care: a guide to practice. Melbourne (Australia): Asumed; 2003. p. 69–86.

[63] Brooks D, Henry J, Leblanc J, et al. Incorporating spirituality into nursing practice. Can Nurse 2005;101(6):22–4.

[64] Sellers SC. The spiritual care meanings of adults residing in the midwest. Nurs Sci Q 2001; 14(3):239–48.

[65] Ornish D. Love and survival. New York: HarperCollins; 1998.

[66] Anselmo J, Kilkmeier LG. Relaxation: the first step to restore, renew and self-heal. In: Dossey BM, Keegan L, Guzzetta CE, editors. Holistic nursing: a handbook for practice. 3rd edition. Gaithersburg (MD): Aspen; 2000. p. 497–535.

[67] Benson H. Timeless healing: the power and biology of belief. New York: Simon & Shuster; 1997.

[68] Lemmer CM. Recognizing and caring for the spiritual needs of clients. J Holist Nurs 2005; 23(3):310–22.

ELSEVIER
SAUNDERS

NURSING
CLINICS
OF NORTH AMERICA

Nurs Clin N Am 42 (2007) 295–307

Creating a Holistic Environment
for Practicing Nurses

Janet Weber, MSN, EdD, RN

*Department of Nursing, Southeast Missouri State University, One University Plaza,
Ms8300, Cape Girardeau, MO 63701, USA*

Today, the practice environment for nurses is uncertain, complex, and ever changing. Factors contributing to this are changes in organizational structures, care delivery models, increased use of unlicensed assistive personnel, increased acuity of illnesses in patients with shorter stays, increased technology, and a shortage of practicing nurses. As the nursing shortage continues, more nurses are leaving the profession. Buerhaus and colleagues [1] predicted that the total number of registered nurses (RNs) would peak in 2007 and decline steadily thereafter as the largest cohort of nurses retires. This attrition should lead to higher nurse/patient care ratios, causing more burnout in nurses who are frustrated because they cannot deliver the knowledgeable compassionate care in which they believe. Although more students are interested in becoming a nurse, the shortage of nursing faculty has caused schools of nursing to accept fewer than 38% of the applications received [2]. Turnover rates for new nursing graduates are 35% to 60% within the first year after graduation [3].

What causes these nurses to leave the profession? New graduate nurses are often unable to handle the intense working environment, advanced technology, and patients with complex health problems. They may feel unprepared to lead a team of health care providers in the management of nursing care for a group of patients. Yet, they are expected to function in this role, which requires them to have a high level of self-awareness, the skills to manage resources, and the ability to lead others [4,5]. In addition, negative relationships that often exist among health care workers may be viewed as a barrier to their dream of practicing as a professional. Loring [6] questioned, "Do nurses really eat their young?" and explained that with fewer nurses and more responsibilities, practicing nurses may view the "new" nurse or student nurse as an extra burden. These nurses often exhibit

E-mail address: jweber@semo.edu

0029-6465/07/$ - see front matter © 2007 Elsevier Inc. All rights reserved.
doi:10.1016/j.cnur.2007.03.003   *nursing.theclinics.com*

a lack of willingness to accept the new person's contribution to clinical care. Staff nurses are frequently the target of verbal abuse by other nurses or physicians, which can have long-term negative effects contributing to lowered nurse job satisfaction, increased absenteeism, and poor patient care [7,8]. This problem contributes to a lowered respect for nursing and a lack of positive regard for nurses in the public arena.

Nurses are often blamed or blame each other for poor patient care, which, in reality, is the result of ineffective work processes promoted. Tucker and Spear [9] found that nurses experience an average of 8.4 work system failures related to medications, orders, supplies, staffing, and equipment within an 8-hour shift. Nursing effectiveness is hindered because of poor health care system processes, which may cause several unnecessary interruptions while a nurse is attempting to provide professional effective nursing care. These work system failures and interruptions lead to job dissatisfaction and frustration.

In some health care settings, nurses may still be viewed as "handmaidens" versus collaborating professional partners with physicians and other health care providers. Hierarchic versus partnering relationships ignore the spirit of the person in today's bureaucratic health care settings. As those in higher positions seek power, a disrespectful and dehumanizing work culture emerges. Wesorick and Shiparski [10] explain that although some nurses are surviving in the workplace setting, it is more important for them to thrive in the workplace. Thriving is more important than surviving, because it is a quality-of-life issue. "Quality exists in the balance of integrated BodyMindSpirit. The human being cannot thrive if there is imbalance" [10]. Conversely, healthy relationships in the workplace strengthen the spirit and give roots to the "BodyMind."

Today, practicing nurses come from four different generations (the veteran generation, the baby boomer generation, generation X, and the millennial generation), which further challenges this complicated health care working environment [11]. Weston [12] explains that tensions arise when nurses from these different generations come together to practice nursing. Veterans tend to follow rules and work hard because they believe that this is what is rewarded by their employer. Conversely, baby boomers question authority and rules and try to transform the status quo. Nurses from generation X are assertive and self-directed and seek job satisfaction, having limited motivation to stay with the same employer. Nurses from the millennial generation are sociable, confident, open-minded, achievement oriented, and interested in contributing to the collective good by volunteering for community services. These various generational attitudes, work habits, and expectations of nurses often lead to misunderstandings and conflict in the workplace.

Despite the emerging transformational leadership theories that are found in the literature, "bureaucratic management" rather than "visionary leadership" persists in health care settings in which nurses practice today. Nurses who possess exemplary patient care skills but lack effective leadership skills continue to be promoted to the position of "Nurse Manager." As a reaction to the complexities of the ever-changing and uncertain health care environment and lack of knowledge of more effective leadership styles, nurse managers and administrators may resort to autocratic controlling styles in an attempt to control versus nurture professional nurses. This type of leadership complicates the nonnurturing environments in which nurses often practice. Nurse managers who rely on orderliness as a problem-solving technique just set up their practice environment for more chaos and unresolved conflict. Traditional forms of nursing leadership used today continue to promote unresolved conflict in the nursing practice environment. "Unresolved conflict always gathers energy and continues to grow in intensity. Always!" [13].

What can be done?

Obviously, there are many factors that contribute to the unhealthy nonnurturing work environments encountered daily by new and experienced nurses. Yet, the American Nurses Association's Bill of Rights for Registered Nurses [14] states: "Nurses have the right to work in an environment that is safe for themselves and their patients." This is usually interpreted as physical safety in regard to proper equipment for lifting and policies that prevent work overload contributing to nurse fatigue and sleep deprivation. The social and emotional safety of registered nurses is equally important, however, so that they are able to provide holistic care to patients. Thus, the physical, emotional, and social environment needs to be addressed. To change this unhealthy practice environment, leaders in clinical practice and educational settings need to begin to view all nurses, including students, new nurses, and aging experienced nurses, as customers who deserve quality practice environments that exceed their expectations.

Implications for clinical practice

First of all, the physical environments in which nurses learn and practice need to be examined. Safety and feasibility to perform one's job and professional responsibilities should be studied and promoted [15]. Physical comfort is essential for practicing nurses if they are to provide this to the patient as their customer.

Malloch and Porter-O'Grady [16] explain that the work environment needs to be studied on how it influences clinical practice. This may be accomplished by examining work flow patterns of the organizational delivery system within the physical system. Assessment of how the structural and organizational environment affects the attitudes, satisfaction, and turnover of practicing nurses needs to be a priority for all nursing administrators. Work that nurses do that does not directly improve patient outcomes needs to be determined and eliminated from the nurse's role. When seeking a place of employment, nurses need to evaluate the environment in which they are planning to work. They should question how the environment is being improved to accommodate the stressful workplace.

Special attention needs to be given to the environment for retaining the baby boomer generation of nurses, who are our most experienced nurses and may provide some stability to the nursing profession. Health care jobs have been identified as top employers for seniors [17]. Some strategies for retaining these seasoned and wise older nurses include flexible part-time work, frequent rest periods, coaches to assist them with the newer technology, respect, and new roles that are less physically demanding (eg, elimination of heavy lifting) [18].

Next, nurses who are leading or being led by traditional forms of leadership need to examine and become more aware of current leadership practice theories. Today, a variety of "newer" leadership theories are evolving in the literature as a response to the quantum-age characteristics of our rapidly changing complex society. Malloch and Porter-O'Grady [13] describe these characteristics as multilateral, multidirectional, relational, interacting, intersecting, and integrating. Four of these newer leadership theories that focus on leader-follower relationships are discussed as potential sources of promoting more nurturing environments for nursing practice. These are Goleman's theory of emotional intelligence [19], clear leadership theory [20], servant leadership [21], and authentic leadership [22].

Goleman's theory of emotional intelligence

This theory focuses on the importance of feelings and self-awareness. Goleman [19] describes "emotional intelligence" as "a learning capability based on emotional intelligence that results in outstanding performance at work." There are four clusters that compose emotional intelligence: self-awareness, self-management, social awareness, and relationship management. Self-awareness is the understanding of one's own feelings and how these feelings affect others and involves ongoing assessment of one's level of self-esteem and self-confidence. Self-management of emotions includes six competencies: control of emotions, trustworthiness, conscientiousness, adaptability, achievement drive, and initiative. Social awareness of people and groups requires empathy, a service orientation, and familiarity with the needs of the organization. Goleman [23] describes eight competencies needed to develop desirable responses in others. These include influence, communication competence, conflict management, visionary leadership, change catalyst, building bonds, collaboration, and teamwork. Some believe that emotional intelligence is more important than IQ or technical abilities in any job [24].

Because of their own insecurities, nurses may tend to act arrogant and put down others in an attempt to seem "right" or more important than fellow colleagues. Negative attitudes and irrational thought processes are futile to the survival of nursing. If nurses are taught self- and social awareness and how to manage oneself and relationships in a positive manner, however, nursing practice environments can be improved. It is clearly understood that nurses must be intelligent and possess a sound knowledge base of nursing and the supporting sciences to provide safe patient care. Possession of this knowledge base without emotional intelligence may jeopardize the process of providing effective patient care with other health team members, however. If a nurse is not aware of how one's actions affect all customers, including patients, nurses, unlicensed assistive personnel, and physicians, unhealthy conflicts may develop.

Nurse administrators and managers need to be aware of low levels of emotional intelligence within themselves and in those nurses who practice in their agency. All nurses should ask themselves if they have weaknesses in any of these clusters and seek assistance as needed to improve their emotional intelligence. Self-help and self-awareness programs should be sought if emotional intelligence tends to be weak. Continuing education on leadership awareness can promote a higher level of emotional intelligence [25].

Clear leadership theory

A leader who is able to practice "clear leadership" is a person who is humble, realizing that leadership is not about him or her but is about helping a group or organization to achieve its goals or increase its effectiveness [20]. When a leader acts in this fashion, a climate of sharing truth, active listening, and working together is promoted. Bushe [20] explains that "interpersonal mush," which is based on fantasies and stories made up about one another, must be eliminated to promote effective productivity. Instead, clear leadership promotes a climate in which all workers are willing to express their own truth and listen to other people's truths. This process promotes understanding and avoids false assumptions. A leader who practices clear leadership is aware of what she or he is feeling, observing, and wanting on a persistent and consistent basis. This leader is able to describe difficult experiences clearly in a manner that is not defensive but causes others to listen. The "clear" leader expresses a sincere curiosity to help others express the truth and uses effective conversation to recognize the best in people and relationships.

Nurse administrators need to share their honest concerns in a humble manner with other nurses, realizing that all nurses provide some type of leadership each day in practice. How often do we continue to witness "games people play" in health care settings in an attempt to gain power or status to overcome one's own insecurities? What would happen if all nurses clearly understood and attempted to practice clear leadership theory? There would be a lot of time left over, because unnecessary gossip that saps energy and time would be reduced. In fact, if focus was given to the truth and humble honesty, energy would be produced. Nurse managers need to find ways to energize their fellow nurses. A videotape that clearly illustrates this concept in active practice is called "Celebrating Our Moments of Excellence" [26]. All nurses working in today's complex and hectic environment may benefit from viewing this videotape to understand the value of truth in practice better.

Servant leadership

Greenleaf [27] explains: "Servant-leadership belongs to a class of leadership philosophies that have the power to bring about dramatic and profound transformation in individuals, their organizations, and the society in which they live." Although the two roles of servant and leader may seem opposite, Greenleaf [27] describes how the two roles can be combined in one real extremely productive person. Greenleaf [27] states: "The servant-leader is servant first. It begins with the natural feeling that one wants to serve. Then conscious choice brings one to aspire to lead. The best test is to ask: Are those being served growing as persons, becoming healthier, wiser, freer, more autonomous, and more likely themselves to become servants?" Spears [28] extracted 10 characteristics of the servant-leader based on Greenleaf's work. These are listening, empathy, healing, awareness, persuasion, conceptualization, foresight, stewardship, commitment to the growth of people, and building of community. A servant-leader is one who does not solve problems in isolation but actively searches for opportunities to build connections to promote creativity and positive human relationships in problem solving. Servant leadership is having a growing impact on a variety of businesses, corporations, churches, universities, health care agencies, and foundations throughout the world [29].

Nursing leaders need to see themselves as servants to those who do the work and to the organization. This servant-leader model enables the nurse leader to see himself or herself in a service role rather than in the traditional hierarchic nurse manager position [13]. Nurse administrators and managers need to ask themselves: "Are the nurses I lead growing as persons, becoming healthier, wiser, freer, and more autonomous with a desire to serve others?" If the answer is "no," they may see their nurses becoming physically and mentally burned out and unhealthy. A study of servant leadership for nurse administrators and staff nurses may open some doors to improve the practice atmosphere. Are those they lead freer and more autonomous or stressed with rigid rules and regulations? Without growing wiser, more autonomous, and freer, nurses are likely to lose their desire to serve others, the very reason why many chose nursing as a career and profession.

Authentic leadership

Authentic leadership is described as positive leadership that is practiced by individuals who have five distinguishing characteristics: purpose, values, heart, relationships, and self-discipline [30,31]. Shirey [32] describes these five characteristics. First the authentic leader continuously reflects and develops a high level of self-awareness in searching for meaning and purpose in life. Next, this leader is highly ethical and values truth. Authentic leaders care about themselves and those they lead. This leader values human relationships. Finally, the authentic leader has a high level of self-discipline that enables him or her to balance his or her personal life and professional life. This type of leadership assumes that a confident, hopeful, optimistic, and resilient leader results in positive behaviors of the leader and followers by building on each person's individual strengths.

Malloch and Porter-O'Grady [13] describe ways to become a fully engaged authentic leader. They describe the authentic leader as one who has a calling for leadership, has integrity, is narcissistic, and tells the whole truth. These principles can easily be applied to nursing leadership as follows. Dedicated leaders usually have an internal calling to "give away one's gifts" in contributing to the world. This calling energizes, affirms, and sustains leaders in times of chaos and conflict. To be authentic, nursing leaders must be their own person in all ways. Attempting to follow the characteristics of others leads to failure as a leader. Instead nurses must ask: "What is my professional identity and what do I stand for?" Box 1 gives helpful questions developed by Malloch and Porter O'Grady [13] that every nurse needs to ask himself or herself. Nurse leaders even need to be a little narcissistic to be healthy and survive. This does not mean that the leader is autocratic but that he or she is assertive, self confident, tenacious, and creative. Nurses need to speak the truth in a caring compassionate manner,

---

Box 1. Questions to ask oneself to be an engaged leader by Malloch and Porter-O'Grady

1. What is important to me? Balance, family, work, success?
2. Do I value stability, innovation, wealth, happiness, humor?
3. What makes me happy, sad, laugh, cry, stressed, calm?
4. Are behaviors that are gregarious, energetic, impulsive, quiet, or shy tolerable to me?
5. How do I treat others? With respect, indifference, selectively?
6. What impact do I want to have on others? To be liked, loved, respected??
7. How do I react to failure? To myself, to others who fail?
8. How do I describe myself? How do others describe me?

Adapted from Malloch K, Porter-O'Grady T. The quantum leader: applications for the new world of work. Sudbury (MA): Jones and Bartlett; 2005. p. 102; with permission.

even when the truth is painful and may cause conflict. This is often seen in the case of the chemically dependent nurse who must be confronted with truthful assistance. It is important that nurses not only listen to others but seriously consider creative ideas from many perspectives. Practicing nurses are extremely creative, and there is nothing worse than having an idea to improve or alter the status quo, only to be met with resistance from a leader. This type of treatment leads to suppressed conflict with severe aftermath consequences.

Continuing education on ways to apply these newer leadership theories in practice is necessary to help nurse managers and administrators learn better ways to lead to promote a healthier practice environment. Self-awareness and team development workshops should be part of all continuing education programs for all nurses and fellow employees in health care agencies. This is especially important for nurse managers who are attempting to lead others and role model acceptable professional behaviors for the development of their nurses and ancillary staff team members. If these newer leadership theories are understood and modeled by nurse mangers, staff nurses may begin to see the benefits and learn to lead others, such as student nurses and new graduate nurses, in this manner, thus promoting a healthier practice environment.

An international effort to transform our current less than acceptable nursing environment into a more nurturing practice environment is the movement for more nursing divisions to seek "magnet status." Magnet status signifies the ability of an agency to attract and retain professional nurses who have high job satisfaction because they can give quality care in their work environment [33]. One of the reasons why magnet-designated hospitals have been successful in the retention of nurses is because of the promotion of processes set in place for "evidence-based practice." Nurses are tired of hearing this so-called "buzz" word; yet, without sound research to support what, how, and where nurses practice, there is little hope of improving the nursing practice environment. Today, there are 223 magnet-recognized organizations in 42 states and 1 in Australia [34]. The "14 forces of magnetism" are listed in Table 1. Within the realm of these 14 forces, McClure and Hinshaw [33] found eight essential factors identified by practicing nurses that need to be present within one's practice environment to be able to provide quality patient care:

Working with other nurses who are clinically competent
Good nurse-physician relationships and communication
Nurse autonomy and accountability
Supportive nurse manager-supervisor
Control over nursing practice and practice environment
Support for education
Adequate nurse staffing
Concern for the patient is paramount

Table 1
Fourteen forces of magnetism

Characteristics	Definition
Quality of nursing leadership	Knowledgeable strong nurse leaders are willing to take risks and advocate for their staff
Organizational structure	Nursing departments are decentralized, with unit-based decision making and strong nurse representation in committees throughout the organization. The nursing leader serves at the executive level of the organization
Management style	Managers involve staff at all levels of the organization. Nurse leaders make an effort to communicate with staff, and staff members feel that their opinions are heard and valued by management
Personnel policies and programs	Salaries and benefits are competitive. There is creative and flexible staffing, with staff involvement. There are many opportunities for promotion in clinical and administrative areas
Professional models of care	Nurses have responsibility, accountability, and authority in their patient care. They coordinate their own support and proper resources from the organization
Quality of care	Nurses believe that they are giving high-quality care to their patients and that their organization sees high-quality care as a priority
Quality improvement	Staff nurses participate in the quality improvement process and believe that it helps to improve patient care within the organization
Consultation and resources	Consultation, including advanced practice nurses and peer support, is available and used
Autonomy	Nurses are allowed and expected to work autonomously, consistent with professional standards as members of a multidisciplinary team
Community and the hospital	Hospitals maintain a strong community presence that includes a variety of long-term outreach programs
Nurses as teachers	Nurses teach in all aspects of their practice
Image of nursing	Nurses are seen as essential to the hospital's delivery of patient care
Interdisciplinary relationships	Relationships are positive with mutual respect by all disciplines
Professional development	Continuing education (orientation, inservices, formal) for professional and personal growth and career development is promoted

Adapted from McClure ML, Hinshaw AS. Magnet hospitals revisited: attraction and retention of professional nurses. Washington (DC): American Nurses Association; 2002. p. 106–7; with permission.

More nurse administrators need to assess for the presence or absence of these 14 forces in their agency. They then need to be proactive and creative in finding ways to develop those forces that may be weak or absent in their own agency. Nurse administrators can find a self-assessment form on-line

[35] if they are considering taking the "magnet journey." Staff nurses may also go to this site to complete a staff nurse questionnaire to assess their practice environment for these forces.

Implications for nursing education

Nursing students are being perceived more and more to health care organizations as an opportunity for recruitment and retention during this time of nursing shortage. Thus, meeting or exceeding the new graduates' expectations is important for nursing education and for employers of new graduates.

How can nursing education meet or exceed these graduates' expectations? First of all, nursing education must prepare new nurses better for what they are about to encounter. This requires not only theory but application of this theory. Painting a rose-colored picture of nursing does not help the new graduate to survive. Educators must be truthful about the research that describes the nonnurturing environment in which nurses often practice. Allowing students to experience reality shock before graduation is necessary to role model ways to deal with conflicts in the workplace setting and to counsel students about healthy methods of how to cope with their feelings. Mawn and Reece [36] describe how the curriculum for the new millennium must be changed to focus on preparing new graduates to possess not only technical skills but managerial and leadership skills.

Some of the leadership characteristics found in the new leadership theories cited in the prior section are self-awareness, participation, patience, values, empathy, and dialog. Although these characteristics may be addressed in baccalaureate nursing programs, the student may not be given an opportunity to witness, apply, or practice these skills and values. Nursing leadership is often "caught" versus "taught" in baccalaureate nursing programs. Yet, the American Association of Colleges of Nursing (AACN) [37] states that leadership is an essential outcome criterion of baccalaureate nursing programs. The nursing shortage often causes a loss of positions for middle mangers and creates more leadership and management activities for staff nurses and new graduates who are at the patient's bedside. Therefore, nursing curricula need to integrate the application of new leadership theories into the student's clinical experiences. The practices of journaling and "post-conferences" can be used to help the student record and discuss observations of "new" versus "old" leadership theories in the practice setting. If new graduates have been introduced to current leadership theories, they learn to recognize the presence of new leadership styles in choosing their practice areas.

Ideally, nursing leaders should all be educated at the master's of nursing science level. With associate degree programs currently producing the highest number of practicing nurses and baccalaureate degree programs producing the second largest number of nurses, however, it is essential for baccalaureate graduates to learn how to implement effective leadership skills to be able to provide the necessary leadership to associate degree–prepared nurses and to assistive unlicensed personnel. Curricula need to be redesigned to teach students the necessary leadership skills they need to promote a healthier work environment for themselves as well as their peers and clients [38]. Young and Urden [39] described a management practicum that prepared new graduates to critically think, embrace change, and collaborate within culturally diverse teams.

A senior-level capstone transitions course can be used to address the real issues of reality shock, burnout, and the nursing shortage. Nursing students ready to graduate can be taught survival skills to deal with conflict effectively, problem solve within groups, and be a change agent in the work setting. Addressing these skills can empower new graduates to have the beginning skills necessary to change practice environments that are less than suitable for practice. The 1999 AACN position statement [40] encourages academia to view itself as a change agent. This requires the nursing education processes to move beyond a reactionary position regarding health care needs and to focus on shaping nursing practice. Baccalaureate students can be taught the beginning processes of how to change the current nonnurturing practice environment.

For example, senior students in a rural midwestern baccalaureate nursing program are required to enroll in a senior leadership course. This course has a clinical component that requires students to collaborate with a baccalaureate-prepared RN (clinical teaching associate) to identify an area for improvement on a specific nursing unit and develop a service learning change project. The AACN [37] also states that service learning can promote the learning of leadership skills. The student applies leadership and change theories to assist nursing staff to improve a part of their practice environment that is hindering them from providing quality patient care. Students research the literature for an evidence base for the change and then educate the staff on what they found. At first, students feel overwhelmed, but by the end of the course, they feel empowered when they see the nursing staff use what they introduced. This type of service learning change project requires close faculty supervision and role modeling to assist students with conflicts encountered and to discuss communication and new emerging leadership skills needed to proceed with the project.

Educators need to inform new graduates about their choices in seeking employment. The characteristics of magnet health care agencies should be explored with senior nursing students to create an awareness of essential factors that promote job satisfaction for nurses. Halfer and Graf [41] found that new graduate nurses were pleased with their overall work experiences in magnet hospitals. Therefore, nurse educators need to support magnet hospitals and health care agencies seeking magnet status.

In summary, until nurse administrators and nurse educators focus on improving the nursing practice environments in which we lead and teach others, it is likely to be extremely difficult for nurses to succeed in providing holistic care to clients. To promote a holistic practice environment for nurses, we need to find creative ways to apply newer leadership theories in practice and education. A heightened self-awareness of our own emotions and how we influence others can promote more positive relationships, and thus a more nurturing practice environment, for nurses of all ages, cultures, and levels of experience.

References

[1] Buerhaus PI, Staiger DO, Auerbach DI. Implications of an aging registered nurse workforce. JAMA 2000;283:2948–54.

[2] National League for Nursing. NLN update. Available at: https://www.nln-updat@ NLN.ORG. 2006;VIII(16). Accessed August 14, 2006.

[3] Beecroft P, Kunzman L, Krozek C. RN internship: outcomes of a one-year pilot program. J Nurs Adm 2001;31(12):575–82.

[4] Gerish K. Still fumbling along? A comparative study of the newly qualified nurse's perception of the transition from student to qualified nurse. J Adv Nurs 2000;32(2):473–80.

[5] Godinez G. Role transition from graduate to staff nurse: a qualitative analysis. J Nurses Staff Dev 1999;15(3):97–110.

[6] Loring CF. Do nurses really eat their young? AWHONN Lifelines 1999;3:47–50.

[7] Rowe MM, Sherlock H. Stress and verbal abusing nursing: do burned out nurses eat their young? J Nurs Manag 2005;13:242–8.

[8] Manderino MA, Berkey N. Verbal abuse of staff nurses by physicians. J Prof Nurs 1997; 13(1):48–55.

[9] Tucker AL, Spear SJ. Operational failures and interruptions in hospital nursing. Health Serv Res 2006;41(3):643–62.

[10] Wesorick B, Shiparski L. Can the human being thrive in the workplace? Grand Rapids (MI): Practice Field Publishing; 1997. p. 5–9.

[11] Sherman R. Leading a multigenerational nursing workforce: issues, challenges, and strategies. Online J Issues Nurs [serial online] 2006;11(2) Manuscript 2. Available at: http:// nursingworld.org/ojin/topic30/tpc30_2.htm. Accessed October 2006.

[12] Weston MJ. Integrating generational perspectives in nursing. Online J Issues Nurs. [serial online] 2006;11(2). Available at: http://nursingworld.org/ojin/topic30/tpc30_1.htm, 2006 Accessed August 18, 2006.

[13] Malloch K, Porter-O'Grady T. The quantum leader: applications for the new world of work. Sudbury (MA): Jones and Bartlett; 2005.

[14] American Nurses Association. American Nurses Association's bill of rights for registered nurses. Adapted by the ANA Board of Directors. Washington, DC: ANA; 2001.

[15] Urlich R, Zimring C. The role of the physical environment in the hospital of the 21st century: a once in a lifetime opportunity. Concord (CA): The Center for Health Design; 2004.

[16] Malloch K, Porter-O'Grady T. Introduction to evidenced based practice. Sudbury (MA): Jones and Bartlett; 2006.

[17] American Association of Retired Persons. AARP Bulletin. September; 2006.

[18] Cipriano P. Editorial: retaining our talent. American Nurse Today 2006;1(2):10.

[19] Goleman D. Working with emotional intelligence. New York: Bantam Books; 1998.

[20] Bushe G. Clear leadership. Palo Alto (CA): Davies-Black Publishing; 2001.

[21] Koch C. Servant leadership: can the bishops learn from Southwest Airlines? America 2004; 191(1):17–9.

[22] George B. The journey to authenticity. Leader to Leader 2004;31:29–35.

[23] Goleman D. An EI theory of performance. In: Cheniss C, Goleman C, editors. The emotionally intelligent workplace. San Francisco (CA): Josey-Bass; 2001. p. 27–44.

[24] Strickland D. Emotional intelligence: the most potent factor in the success equation. J Nurs Adm 2000;30(3):112–7.

[25] Vitello-Cicciu JM. Exploring emotional intelligence: implications for nurse leaders. J Nurs Adm 2002;32(4):203–9.

[26] Wright D. Celebrating our moments of excellence [videotape]. . Minneapolis (MN): Creative Health Care Management; 2002.

[27] Greenleaf R. The servant leader within: a transformative path. Mahwah (NJ): Paulist Press; 2003.

[28] Spears LC. The understanding and practice of servant-leadership. In: Spears LC, Lawrence M, editors. Practicing servant leadership: succeeding through trust, bravery, and forgiveness. San Francisco (CA): Josey-Bass; 2004. p. 9–24.

[29] Spears LC, Lawrence M. Practicing servant leadership: succeeding through trust, bravery, and forgiveness. San Francisco (CA): Josey-Bass; 2004.

[30] George B. Authentic leadership: rediscovering the secrets to creating lasting value. San Francisco (CA): Josey-Bass; 2003.

[31] Luthans F, Aviolio B. Authentic leadership development. In: Cameron KS, Dutton JE, Quin RE, editors. Positive organizational scholarship. San Francisco (CA): Barrett-Koehler; 2003. p. 241–58.

[32] Shirey MR. Fostering leadership through collaboration. Authentic leadership: foundation of a healthy work environment. Reflections on nursing leadership. Honor Society of Nursing Sigma Theta Tau International Web site. Available at: http://www.nursingsociety.org/RNL/Current/features/features5.htlm. Accessed October 2, 2006.

[33] McClure ML, Hinshaw AS. Magnet hospitals revisited: attraction and retention of professional nurses. Washington, DC: American Nurses Association; 2002.

[34] ANCC Magnet Recognition Program Web site. Recognizing excellence in nursing services. 2006. Available at: http://nursingworld.org/ancc/magnet/index.html. Accessed November 22, 2006.

[35] Available at: http://nursingworld.org/ancc/magnet/index.htlm.

[36] Mawn B, Reece S. Reconfiguring a curriculum for the new millennium: the process of change. J Nurs Educ 2000;39(3):101–8.

[37] American Association of Colleges of Nursing. 1998 Essentials of baccalaureate education. Washington, DC: AACN; 1998.

[38] Young J, Urden LD, Wellman DS, et al. Management curriculum design. Nurse Educ 2004; 29(1):41–4.

[39] Young J, Urden LD. Student stakeholders impact redesign for management curriculum. Nurse Educ 2004;29(6):251–5.

[40] American Association of Colleges of Nursing. Nursing education's agenda for the 21st agenda [position statement]. Washington, DC: AACN; 1999.

[41] Halfer D, Graf E. Graduate nurse perceptions of the work experience. Nurs Econ 2006;24(3): 150–5.

NURSING
CLINICS
OF NORTH AMERICA

ELSEVIER
SAUNDERS

Nurs Clin N Am 42 (2007) 309–333

Teaching Holistic Nursing: The Legacy of Nightingale

Margaret O'Brien King, PhD, RNBC, AHNBC[a],*,
Marie F. Gates, PhD, RN[b]

[a]Department of Nursing, College of Social Sciences, Health, and Education,
Xavier University, 3800 Victory Parkway, Cincinnati, OH 45207-7351, USA
[b]Western Michigan University, Bronson School of Nursing,
1903 West Michigan Avenue, Kalamazoo, MI 49008, USA

Nursing has a lengthy record of meeting the needs of humanity and has been the vanguard in providing care and comfort to those who are ill and dying. In addition, nursing has provided education to preserve the health of the public. Recognizing the need for these services, nursing has honored differences in culture, religion, values, economics, and individual needs and concerns. Historical evidence of nursing meeting client needs is apparent through the work of Nightingale, Wald, Sanger, and Breckinridge. These nursing leaders, among many others, made an impact on society by considering not only the physical component of the person but also the interconnectedness of the body, mind, and spirit of every individual.

During the past 30 years, nursing has been moving away from a physiologic-scientific focus toward a nursing-caring-healing model. Watson [1] describes this movement as a paradigm shift from nurses helping doctors practice medicine to nurses practicing the distinct art and science of nursing. This change in focus has directed nursing's return to the philosophy and teachings of Florence Nightingale, who emphasized that the nurse must use the hands, heart, and head in creating healing environments to care for the patient's body, mind, and spirit.

Research suggests a growing public interest in holistic nursing and national surveys concur that health care consumers are seeking a holistic approach to their health care [2]. Patients desire a health care practitioner who listens and is caring [2]. These practitioners are often identified as holistic, which generally means that the health care practitioner considers the whole

* Corresponding author.
E-mail address: kingm@xavier.edu (M.O. King).

0029-6465/07/$ - see front matter © 2007 Elsevier Inc. All rights reserved.
doi:10.1016/j.cnur.2007.03.007
nursing.theclinics.com

person, including physical, mental, emotional, and spiritual aspects. Dossey and Dossey [3] point out that patients may consider the health care professional unscientific if the elements of mind, soul, and spirit are not honored along with the physical while caring for the patient. Because patients are holistic beings, it is nursing's responsibility to be attentive to society's requests and needs for holistic nurses.

Holistic nursing

Nursing as a profession has long espoused the use of the term holistic and has included the term in nursing literature and practice. Holistic nursing has often been the prominent concept in narratives describing nursing education programs and standards of practice, policies, and regulations [4]. The American Holistic Nurses' Association (AHNA) defines holistic nursing in this manner: "Holistic nursing embraces all nursing which has as its goal enhancement of healing the whole person from birth to death"[5].

The Nightingale legacy

Beginning in the nineteenth century, Florence Nightingale wrote in her text, *Notes on Nursing*, that nursing's role is to "put the patient in the best condition for nature to act upon him" [6]. In other words, nursing is to assist the patient to a return to a state of health or to simply preserve the patient's health by preventing or curing disease [7]. Nightingale believed that health was not merely the absence of disease, but extended to the individual's capacity to live life to the fullest [8]. This is consistent with the philosophy of the twenty-first century that health is not simply the absence of disease but maximizing one's quality of life and potential [9]. Although Nightingale struggled for full meaning of questions concerning human existence, she was able to understand that healing required deliberate and full attention to the body, mind, spirit, and environment [10]. Nightingale was well aware that the concept of health was not a separate component distinct from relationships with the people and the world in which we live [11]. She believed that healing is an active process of recuperating from an illness, repair of something broken, restoration of oneself to a former state, and transformation of the mind, body, and soul on the journey to becoming more complete [12,13]. The healing experience may or may not involve curing [14].

It is imperative that nurses continue Nightingale's philosophy of holistic nursing. If nursing ignores Nightingale's philosophy of holistic nursing, patients do not receive the care they are requesting. Patients expect compassionate experts focused on the whole person, nothing less. Through Nightingale's legacy, nursing can meet that expectation. Her philosophy included nurse self-care, nursing art, science, related theories, research, and ethics [15]. Nightingale demonstrated in her work and discussed in her writings that her major tenet was healing—the process of bringing together all aspects of the individual body, mind, and spirit to achieve and maintain integration and balance. She made a distinction between healing and curing. She believed that healing was always possible, whereas curing a disease might not always occur. Curing was only the removal of the signs and symptoms of disease. This removal of the signs and symptoms of disease might not stop or resolve a person's disease or distress because it involved only one dimension, the physical. Curing may not consider the whole person—body, mind, and spirit. Healing seeks ways for the person to find harmony and balance in life, family, and community. Healing is part of the process of living and dying; it addresses the body, mind, and spirit of the person. Nightingale further saw the patient as the interpreter of his or her own experience capable of self-care practices, whereas the nurse was the person who assisted the patient in the healing journey. Because Nightingale [16] believed that healing involves both the internal and external environment, she emphasized that nurses are responsible for creating a healing environment through their therapeutic presence with the patient. "We must not talk to them or at them but with them."

Being mindful of the influence of the external physical environment on the person, Nightingale instituted the use of color, light, music, pets, relaxation, nutrition, exercise, and flowers to provide a healing external environment. Nightingale [6] emphasized that "The effect in sickness of beautiful objects, of variety of objects, and especially of brilliancy of color, is hardly at all appreciated." She relates that "people say that effect is only on the mind. It is no such thing. The effect is on the body too...Variety of form and brilliancy of color in the objects presented to patients are actual means of recovery" [6]. Nightingale [6], relating a personal experience, stated, "I remember (in my own case) a nosegay of wild flowers being sent me, and from that moment recovery becoming more rapid. The effect of music upon the sick has been scarcely at all noticed...wind instruments, including the human voice, and stringed instruments, capable of continuous sound, have generally a beneficent effect" [6]. All of this speaks to the role of the nurse "to put the patient in the best condition for nature to act upon him" [6] and to combine "the proper use of fresh air, light, warmth, cleanliness, quiet and the proper selection and administration of diet—all at the least expense of vital power to the patient" [6]. Further discussion of the influence of the environment is discussed when Nightingale sates when it comes to variety, "I incline to think that the majority of cheerful cases is to be found among those patients who are not confined to one room, whatever their suffering, and that the majority of depressed cases will be seen among those subjected to a long monotony of objects about them" [6]. For those who might be alone, Nightingale [6] wrote, "A small pet animal is often an excellent companion for the sick, for long chronic cases especially. A pet bird in a cage is sometimes the only pleasure of an invalid confined for years to the same room. If he can feed and clean the animal himself, he ought always to be encouraged to do so".

For the nurse to be an effective caregiver, Nightingale [17] wrote in her letter of 1878 to a group of nursing students about the importance of self-care and to use personal reflection to become a good nurse. She suggested that the students look closely into the philosophy and ethic of caring for and healing of self. Slater and colleagues [18] further affirm Nightingale's beliefs by asserting that becoming a holistic nurse requires an understanding of how to be present to all facets of the patient and this genuine presence demands first that the nurse be present to all aspects of him or herself. Jonas and colleagues [14] concur with Nightingale and Slater and colleagues that the nurse needs to be healed first. To provide maximal healing presence, nurses need to maintain a degree of wholeness and well-being themselves through self-care and reflection.

In summary, Nightingale describes the role of the nurse as one who is able to put the patient in the best possible condition for nature to act, thereby facilitating the laws of nature. The nurse is able to facilitate this process by changing the environment, internal and external, to best meet the needs of the patient's body, mind, and spirit. Nightingale believed that people were multifaceted, composed of physical, mental, social, and spiritual elements. The spiritual component is not addressed overtly in Nightingale's writings but it is an assumed component because of her profound discussions of her own spirituality and its impact on her work, her way of life, and her relationships with others [9].

Teaching nursing students to become holistic nurses

Over the time since Nightingale first influenced the major change in nursing, there have been many changes in care dictated through advances in science and technology and the nurse has journeyed on this technological path, at times veering away from the philosophic foundation established by Nightingale. Now in the twenty-first century, there is increased recognition and appreciation for the care of the whole person—body, mind, and spirit—as prescribed by Nightingale. Nursing education must follow the example set forth by Nightingale and teach students to become holistic nurses.

By embracing the philosophy of nursing's founder, Florence Nightingale, nursing can continue to meet society's needs by preparing holistic practitioners. This article discusses the impact of the consumer's request for holistic practitioners and nursing's response with the preparation of holistic nurses. Faculty from two schools endorsed by the American Holistic Nurses' Credentialing Commission (AHNCC) discuss ways in which their respective schools have incorporated holistic nursing in their curricula. Faculty at one school, Western Michigan University (WMU) located in Kalamazoo, Michigan, adopted holistic nursing as one of its primary conceptual bases. As a result, faculty members were aware at the school's inception of that focus. Faculty at a second school, Xavier University

(XU) located in Cincinnati, Ohio, decided to incorporate holistic principles some time after the school was formed. This article provides a glimpse of how the schools embraced and incorporated holistic nursing into their programs. It concludes with strategies to promote that incorporation and to overcome barriers to inclusion of holistic nursing in the curriculum.

A holistic nursing curriculum

A holistic curriculum is focused not just on the physical but also on the emotional and spiritual needs of patients. "Holistic nursing draws on nursing knowledge, theories, research, expertise, intuition, and creativity" [19] to guide nurses in becoming therapeutic partners with clients in strengthening the clients' responses to facilitate the healing process and achieve wholeness. Consideration of the whole person is integrated throughout the curriculum. The concept of healing the whole person from birth to death is emphasized, with the nurse as the facilitator in the healing process. Communication is emphasized for the nurse to be present with the client and honor the client's personal experiences related to their health, health beliefs, and values. Experiences are provided to assist students to become therapeutic partners with individuals, families, and communities. "Practicing holistic nursing requires nurses to integrate self-care, self-responsibility, spirituality, and reflection in their lives" [19]. "Self-responsibility leads the nurse to a greater awareness of the interconnectedness of all individuals and their relationships to the human and global community, and permits nurses to use this awareness to facilitate healing" [3]. Students are introduced to opportunities to begin the life- long practice of "know thyself." For the graduate nurse to facilitate the patient through the healing journey, students are offered opportunities to integrate self-care and self-responsibility, explore their own spirituality, and reflect on their lives. All of these activities assist students in increasing their understanding and appreciation of all people and a deeper awareness of their relationship to the overall human and global community. All of this heightened attentiveness assists the student in becoming a more effective therapeutic partner in facilitating the healing process. The holistic nurse is the professional who becomes one with the patient through transpersonal communication and is with the patient as the client proceeds along his or her journey. Lack of presence with the patient impedes the patient's progress with his or her journey. Nightingale emphasized that nursing is putting the patient in the best possible position for nature to act by focusing on the interconnectedness of the mind, body, and spirit. This goal can only be accomplished through holistic nursing.

Identifying characteristics of a holistic nursing curriculum

The holistic curriculum prepares the nurse to be well versed in the art of nursing, not just the science of nursing. The holistic nurse views the patient through a different lens than a non-holistic nurse. The patient is seen through the nurse's exposure to human-to-human care and not just understood through the science of nursing. The nurse is prepared to "help persons gain a higher degree of harmony within the mind, body, and soul which generates self-knowledge, self-reverence, self-healing, and self-care processes while allowing increasing diversity" [1]. Spirituality and nursing presence are emphasized as essential elements in the practice of holistic nursing. It has been suggested that these two concepts are paramount to holistic nursing [20,21]. To practice nursing presence, spirituality, the manifestation of a person's essence, is primary [22,23]. Rankin and DeLashmutt [24] found in their study with nursing students that students believed that "spirituality is a foundational requisite of nursing presence; it is the backbone to nursing presence".

Impact of the holistic nurse

Through the holistic nurse's presence, the holistic nurse enters into the experience of the patient, and the patient enters into the nurse's experience [25]. This transpersonal human caring experience strengthens and provides wisdom to the healing journey for both individuals. The nurse is exposed to the process of self-assessment and self-healing. This exposure assists the nurse in recognizing his or her strengths and weaknesses and purpose and meaning in life. Through self-reflection, the nurse develops trust in his or her intuition and is able to move into a higher level of awareness [26]. This awareness facilitates the nurse to see more and be more with the patient. With this awareness, the nurse is able to be more fully present in the moment to assist the patient with the healing journey.

Building a holistic curriculum

To begin the process of defining a curriculum as holistic, one might want to examine the AHNA Standards of Holistic Nursing Practice. These standards can be used as a template for the development of course objectives and teaching strategies. The AHNA Standards of Holistic Practice describe the professional activities, knowledge, and performance that are expected from a holistic nurse [19]. Mariano discusses the AHNA Standards of Holistic Nursing Practice elsewhere in this issue.

Educators can examine curriculum content related to the five core values and standards under each core when developing course content. An example of determining where core values and standards may fall in specific courses is found in Box 1. The core value discussed is core value 4: holistic communication, therapeutic environment, and cultural diversity. The table identifies a few of the many nursing activities that could be implemented to facilitate learning experiences to meet the standards of this core. These standards and nursing activities are from the AHNA Standards of Holistic Nursing Practice: Guidelines for Caring and Healing [19].

Box 1. Core value and standards with samples of nursing activities for inclusion in courses; Core Value 4: Holistic communication, therapeutic environment, and cultural diversity

Holistic communication standards:
Awareness of communication challenges
    Activities: develop communication skills, active problem solving strategies
Increase therapeutic and cultural competence
    Activities: use cultural health care assessment, respect for cultural rituals
Explore deeper meaning, purpose, inner strengths, and connections
    Activities: spiritual assessment tool, strategies to nurture the spirit
Recognize communication and awareness of individuals is continuously evolving
    Activities: care of the body, mind, spirit; relaxation techniques; body, mind, healing processes
Respect person's health trajectory
    Activities: respect decision for use of traditional, CAM (complementary/alternative modalities)

Environment standards:
Promote healing environments
    Activities: use nursing process to prevent problems, reduce hazards, manipulate to foster health
Create organizations that value sacred space
    Activities: join professional associations, personal and professional development
Integrate holistic principles, standards, policies, and procedures in relation to environmental safety
    Activities: awareness of environmental space and hazards
Recognize ecosystem is a prior determining condition
    Activities: environmental assessment
Promote social networks and healing environments
    Activities: social justice ethic, assess personal environmental stress

Cultural diversity standards:
Assess and incorporate person's cultural practices, values, beliefs
    Activities: cultural health assessment, communication skills
Use appropriate community resources
Open-minded about cultural differences
Assess for discriminatory practices
Identify discriminatory health practices
    Activities: examine personal value and beliefs, make decision that support ethical and moral principles

Data from Frisch NC, Dossey BM, Guzzetta CE, et al. AHNA standards of holistic nursing practice. Gaithersburg (MD): Aspen Publishers, Inc.; 2000; with permission.

Graduates of a holistic nursing curriculum

A holistic curriculum prepares students to become nurses who facilitate the patient's healing process. Students are prepared to apply the art and science of nursing by drawing on nursing knowledge, theories, expertise, intuition, and creativity to guide them in becoming a therapeutic partner with the patient and integrating self-care in their lives.

A holistic nursing program prepares nurses to be present with their patients no matter what the specialty area of practice. The nurse must place equal emphasis on technical skills, broad base of knowledge, and therapeutic presence. A model of this dynamic interaction is presented in Fig. 1. The model depicts three eclipses overlapping: holistic nursing knowledge, holistic therapeutic presence, and holistic nursing skills. The intersection of the circles exemplifies the importance of all three components of the healing relationship that represent the cognitive, affective, and psychomotor domains. One aspect of holistic nursing is not more important than the others. All are equally compelling. When all three domains interact with each other, there is greater impact. Students gain an understanding of the meaning of healing and what they can do every day to facilitate healing not only with the patient but also in themselves. Students become exceedingly aware of how their presence influences the healing journey of the patient.

The model also depicts healing evolving from the interrelated dynamics of the patient's and the nurse's body-mind-sprit. The healing environment can be developed through this dynamic presence of the nurse's trying to

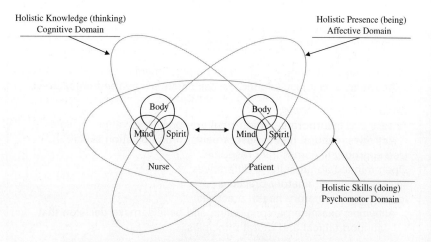

Courtesy of Xavier University Department of Nursing, Cincinnati, Ohio; with permission.

Fig. 1. Holistic presence, holistic thinking, and holistic doing in the holistic healing relationship.

connect with another. It is the nurse who is given the most sacred opportunity to walk with the patient on their healing journey so that the patient is not alone at the defining moment of healing. When the holistic nurse enters into the profound nurse–patient relationship, the nurse is interconnected with the patient. As O'Brien [27] states, at this moment the nurse is walking on sacred ground and neither is the same afterward.

The role of complementary and alternative therapies

Currently there is an increasing interest in the use of complementary alternative modalities (CAM) and increasing acceptance by the public [28,29]. The National Institutes of Health's Office of Alternative Medicine defines CAM as a group of diverse medical and health care systems, practices, and products that are not presently considered to be part of conventional medicine. The list of CAM changes continually as those therapies that are proven to be safe and effective become adopted into conventional health care and new approaches to health care emerge [29]. The public finds holistic practices, CAM, and holistic practitioners appealing because these practices and practitioners offer approaches that emphasize self-healing. Self-healing gives patients some degree of control over their health along with individualized, holistic, and high-touch care, and a potential for reduction in side effects [2]. Holistic practitioners emphasize healing rather than curing a disease by focusing on the interrelationship of the patient's body, mind, and spirit. This focus is based on a total commitment to the practice of good health care, whether its origins are traditional therapies or CAM [30].

The holistic nurse may wish to have more therapeutic options available to assist the patient on his or her journey but these therapeutics are not the sole criterion that characterizes the nurse as holistic. The learning of CAM is secondary to the broad base of knowledge and therapeutic presence when preparing a holistic practitioner. Knowledge and awareness of CAM are important for the nurse to engage in conversation with patients but are not critical elements to becoming a holistic nurse. It is a misnomer when one considers that to be holistic one has to simply embrace the many integrative modalities that many Americans are now using.

CAM is a necessary part of the curriculum but only as a tool to assist the patient in his or her journey. Introduction to a variety of these modalities, the evidence base for these modalities, and strategies to implement these modalities are important for inclusion in the curriculum. Because 62% of Americans at this time are using CAM [31], nurses must learn about these modalities and their use to meet the changing needs of patients. Such knowledge helps nurses assist patients with wise choices.

Today's nurse must integrate the best of traditional therapies with nontraditional therapies through a caring–healing focus to empower individuals on their healing journey. In other words, nursing must return to its roots and follow the traditions of Florence Nightingale by implementing holistic nursing care.

Complementary alternative modalities and therapeutic presence

A focus group of nurse educators at the 2003 AHNA Conference discussed the increasing number of nursing schools offering CAM in their programs [32]. The importance of nurse self-care, the instruction of patients in self-care, the importance of CAM, and the effect of using CAM within traditional health care services have also been well documented [4,33–35].

Along with the use of CAM and the importance of nurse and patient self-care, presence or being was also found to be a key point in the holistic process by the focus group. The focus group found that presence is an essential nursing intervention, not always addressed, noted, or recorded. Patients often assume the nurse to be an expert technician; anecdotes from patients often do not address or emphasize the skilled (doing) and knowledgeable (thinking) care of the nurse but simply speak of the nurse's presence and compassion. Patients may not call it therapeutic presence but this presence is identified by comments from the patient, such as, "the nurse was there," "was with me," "held my hand," "comforted me," explained everything to me," "was kind," "sensed my embarrassment," "made me laugh," and "supported me throughout my illness" (similar to the nurse assisted me with my journey). Being present with the patient on his or her journey energizes the nurse and the patient. Being present with the patient offers the nurse an opportunity to experience the heartfelt passion that holistic nursing can offer.

Two schools' experiences

The experiences of WMU and XU provide a complementary view of how holistic nursing was incorporated within their programs. WMU offered holistic nursing from its inception; XU integrated holistic nursing into an existing program.

Western Michigan University

The nursing program at WMU Bronson School of Nursing (BSON) was developed in 1994 with the goal of meeting current and emerging health care needs of society. The original core aspects of the curriculum included relationship-centered care, holistic nursing care, and community-based care. Through the generous support of the Bronson and Borgess Hospitals (the two major hospitals within the city), the Fetzer Institute, the Irving S. Gilmore Foundation, and the W.K. Kellogg Foundation, the BSON established this program and maintained its major tenets throughout a recent curriculum revision.

With the assistance of consultants, notably Jean Watson, faculty decided on a praxis framework emphasizing the cognitive, affective, and psychomotor domains. The program objectives stated that the curriculum was designed to prepare professional nurses who promoted self-care, health, and harmony throughout the lifespan, and reached out in response to the needs of the community. Students were expected to identify patterns influencing health, well-being, and illness within individuals, families, groups, and communities.

The initial curriculum introduced the holistic philosophy and self-care components in its first courses for both the pre-licensure and registered nurse (RN) completion students. The American Nurses Association (ANA) standards and the AHNA standards served as the ethical foundation for current and revised courses and in the development of clinical practice evaluation instruments for the undergraduate program.

Box 2 presents an overview of the key elements included in the BSON curriculum plan. Dossey's holistic nursing book is an essential textbook that was introduced early and continued throughout the other courses [36]. Experiences throughout the program are planned to incorporate holistic nursing components throughout the student's course of study. Table 1 presents the correspondence of selected holistic content as offered in courses throughout the undergraduate curriculum at WMU BSON. Schools of nursing may be providing more of a holistic essence to their programs than they realize. When the WMU BSON developed its original matrix of holistic component with delineation of content and where taught, it helped faculty determine how consistently the content was provided. For example, presentation of CAM includes presentation of specific modalities for use by students, identification of evidence base for those modalities through the research course, and evaluation of the use of modalities in the clinical practice arena. The presence of the Holistic Health Care Department within the College of Nursing allowed for more effective collaboration between nursing and holistic health care in teaching and evaluating that specific component in the curriculum. The move of the college to the new building in which a wellness laboratory was planned contributed to the efficacy of teaching of health care modalities.

Throughout the BSON nursing program students work in partnership with others as they learn to incorporate ways of improving their knowledge and practice of caring in patient–practitioner, community–practitioner, and practitioner–practitioner relationships. The Fetzer Institute was able to support workshops offered in tandem with the community to enable holistic content to be offered not only to students but also to practitioners within the community. Early in the inception of the program the BSON had two full-fledged certified holistic nurses, but other career options for these nurses led them to leave the school. The commitment of the faculty to continue the holistic framework led them to continue their own education in holistic nursing. The faculty met on a regular basis to gain expertise and

Box 2. Western Michigan University Bronson School of Nursing overview of curriculum plan

Mission:
BSON is rooted in relationship-centered interdisciplinary care, evidence-based practice, and holism. The curriculum is designed to prepare professional nurses who promote self-care, health, and harmony throughout the lifespan and reach out in response to the needs of the community

Core objectives
Provide holistic, caring, and culturally sensitive nursing care for communities, groups, and individuals
Develop community health partnerships with clients and other health providers to shape health policy
Promote health and prevent disease
Analyze and apply nursing research and scholarly inquiry to inform professional practice
Accept responsibility and accountability for behavior consistent with the profession's code of ethics and standards for professional practice
Use critical thinking to guide professional practice
Use effective human technological communication in professional practice to enhance the health and well-being of diverse individuals, families, and communities

Courses
Sophomore courses
NUR 2200. Foundations of nursing and critical thinking
NUR 2210. Nursing therapeutics I
NUR 2220 Health assessment throughout the lifespan
NUR 2300 Concepts of health & wellness in nursing practice
NUR 2310 Wellness care of the elder
Junior courses
NUR 3200 Wellness and health promotion in families
NUR 3210 Care of families and children with alterations in health status
NUR 3220 Health care ethics
NUR 3300 Nursing therapeutics II
NUR 3310 Care of adults with alterations in health status
NUR 3320 Research in nursing practice
NUR 3330 Informatics for health
Senior courses
NUR 4200 Psychiatric mental health nursing
NUR 4210 Nursing care of patient with complex conditions
NUR 4310 Populations-based nursing

Courtesy of Western Michigan University, Bronson School of Nursing, Kalamazoo, Michigan; with permission.

Table 1
Comparison of selected holistic content with specific courses

Holistic content	Placement and examples of topics and experiences
AHNA and ANA ethical components core holistic values	All courses with clinical components, concentrated emphasis in health care ethics course
Holistic philosophy	Introductory nursing course for pre-licensure and RN completion courses, community health and wellness course
Self-care	All nursing courses; expectation that self-care principles will be defined in journals and plans for all courses
Holistic modalities, CAM (complementary/alternative modalities)	Selected modalities taught and practiced in concepts of health and wellness in nursing practice; therapeutics I and II courses; identified in nursing care plans throughout clinical courses; relationship of medications with modalities in pharmacology course
Evidence base for practice for holistic nursing and CAM	Nursing research course; nursing informatics course
Communication	Process recordings in well elder course, other clinical courses; initially content in critical thinking and therapeutics I course; higher-level content in psychiatric mental health nursing and nursing therapeutics II; monitoring of levels throughout all clinical practice courses, including care of adults, well and ill individuals and families, clients who have complex conditions
Community health and partnerships	Concepts of health and wellness and population-based courses; community projects in well elder, concepts of health and wellness, teaching projects, community projects; management/leadership projects
Human diversity, spirituality, and global health care	All courses, with emphasis in population-based nursing, health care, ethics course
Health care systems and policy	Critical thinking and foundations of nursing, nursing management leadership courses; tracking of content throughout program by papers, iwebfolio

Courtesy of Western Michigan University, Bronson School of Nursing, Kalamazoo, Michigan; with permission.

foundations for the teaching of holistic nursing. Currently, one faculty member has certification as a holistic nurse. Several other faculty members are preparing themselves to take the certification examination also. Although the director did not secure her own certification, she has been active with AHNA in presenting several workshops at the annual meetings.

The current curriculum has been revised but continues to include the program of study leading to infusion of holistic nursing in the curriculum. The major hospital systems in the community support the existence of the holistic framework and have holistic or integrative care centers within their institutions. The environment in which WMU exists provides support for the teaching of holistic nursing.

Xavier University

The XU nursing program was not deliberately developed to be a holistic nursing curriculum. It evolved from an existing curriculum plan and was identified as holistic after faculty completed a comprehensive review process. This review process was initiated after they were contacted by the AHNCC for consideration as an endorsed program.

As all nurse educators are well aware, accrediting bodies necessitate that curriculum incorporate the overriding mission of the institution. The holistic curriculum thus began with the mission. The mission of XU emphasizes excellence in academics as found in most institutions of higher learning, and also attention to the student as an individual and a sense of the whole person—body, mind, and spirit.

XU's mission statement strongly reflects the key elements found in the holistic nurse: intellectual skills necessary for a full life as a consumer in society; critical attention to the underlying philosophic and theologic implications of issues; a world view that is oriented to responsible action and recognition of the intrinsic value of natural and human values; an understanding and communication of moral and religious values through personal concern and lived witness and by precept and instruction; and a sense of the whole person—body, mind, and spirit. The university mission statement is complemented by the college and nursing department's mission statement.

XU graduates are well grounded in philosophy, ethics, nursing theories, research, holism, self-care, health promotion, sense of meaning, and various modalities. Therapeutic presence, the most powerful tool for healing, is emphasized as an essential component of every nursing action. Graduates of Xavier's programs realize the nurse is an instrument of healing. Opportunities for exploration of spirituality are offered throughout the curriculum and attentiveness to one's spirit is emphasized as basic to the healing interaction with another. Recognition of another's free choice is of paramount importance in facilitating a client's transition. New graduates repeatedly report they recognize their holistic approach to patient care is uniquely apparent when compared with graduates from other programs.

Initially XU offered one curriculum in nursing preparing RNs to earn a Bachelor of Science in Nursing degree. To better meet the needs of the community, the XU faculty was charged by the President to develop a new curriculum to prepare undergraduate students to earn the Bachelor of Science in Nursing degree. At this point, important elements emerged that led to the course of action that evolved into the aforementioned curriculum. With this new charge, faculty began the process of meeting, discussing, and debating issues that were important to the new undergraduate curriculum. For the change to take place particular elements facilitated readiness. These elements are as follows:

One faculty member developed an interest in learning about CAM, whereas some faculty members were skeptical.

Faculty began discussing the impact of CAM on transpersonal communication and therapeutic presence.

Faculty began to be aware that it was important to find like-minded colleagues when engaging in discussions about the use of CAM.

Faculty learned to speak gently and kindly with those colleagues who were not at the same acceptance level with the use of CAM to continue meaningful dialogue.

Five holistic elective courses were initiated emphasizing the use of integrative therapies in the care of the older adult, pain management, and self-care. The elective courses became very popular with nursing and non-nursing majors.

A faculty member who had completed research on nurses' knowledge and use of complementary therapies discussed her findings through a continuing education presentation for faculty and alumni. This discussion was given great reviews.

Faculty members who were enthused about the use of CAM were invited to discuss their experience and research with freshman nursing classes.

Two tenured faculty members became certified as holistic nurses (HNC).

The two HNCs taught at the sophomore level and incorporated discussion of CAM and evidence-based research in their courses.

As all of these activities materialized, the chair of the program received a letter from AHNCC inquiring if the program was interested in applying for endorsement as a holistic nursing program. This inquiry was the stimulus that initiated the review of the program resulting in the identification of XU's program as holistic.

Even though the program had not used the AHNA's Core Values and Standards of Holistic Nursing in its development, these concepts were found to be present in the overlying philosophy and courses of the program. Faculty examined their courses and determined which of the values and standards were included. They identified which course objectives addressed those issues. This review gave all faculty a clear and comprehensive understanding of when and in what courses specific elements of holistic nursing were presented. An example of the model used for this review is found in Table 2.

Although holistic nursing is not defined as CAM, the complementary modality of healing touch was the catalyst to the understanding of the phenomena of transpersonal communication, therapeutic presence, spirituality, and the many other components of holistic nursing. The discussion of the use and value of healing touch stimulated much conversation, skeptical and supportive. The concept of healing touch was often the focus of spirited discussions (pro and con). The faculty, who became interested in learning and

Table 2
Concepts addressed in holistic nursing practice within selected nursing courses according to course objectives at Xavier University

BSN Program	NURS 130	NURS 132	NURS 224	NURS 225	NURS 230	NURS 231	NURS 360	NURS 361	NURS 370	NURS 372	NURS 373	NURS 410	NURS 450
PART I: Nurse-focused concepts													
I. Professional education & personal development	1,3,6	3	3	4	1	—	1,2,6	1,3,7,8	1	—	8	1,7	1,4
II. Community & global involvement	1,3,6	1,2,3,4	3	4	2	—	1,2	3,9	3	1	—	—	2,6
PART II: Client/patient-focused concepts													
III. Caring for the whole client/patient & family/ significant others	—	2	1,2,4,5	1,2,3	1,2,3	5	1–5	1–5	—	1,5,7	1,2,3,7	2,25	1–4
IV. Health education & mutual decision-making	—	2,4	1,2,5	1,2,3	1,2,3	2,4	1,4,6	1,4,5,6	—	All	All	—	3,4,6
V. Cultural care	—	1,2,3,4	1,3,4	1,2,3	1,3	2,5	22–5	2,4,5,6	—	4	6	—	1,2,4,6
VI. Health promotion	—	1,4	1,2,3,4,5	1,2,3	1,2	4	1,2	2,8	—	—	—	—	3,4,6
VII. Self-care	—	3,4	1,2,3,4,5	4	1	2	3,4	4,5	—	All	—	—	3,4
VIII. Spiritual care	—	2	1,2,3,4,5	1,2,3	—	5	2,3,4	4,5	—	—	—	—	2,3,4
IX. Care of the environment	All	—	1,2,3	3,4	—	1	3,4,5	4,5,6	—	—	5	—	2,3,4
X. Research/ theory	All	—	3,4	—	1	3	1,2	2,8	1,2,3,4	—	—	8	1,2
XI. Nursing process	All	—	1,2,3,4,5	1,2,3,4	1	2	3,4,5	4,5,6	2	—	5	2,3	3,5
XII. Nursing theory	All	—	3	—	1	2	1,4,2	2,8	2,3	—	—	—	1,2,4

Courtesy of Xavier University Department of Nursing, Cincinnati, Ohio; with permission.

experiencing healing touch, began to discuss with others the impact this modality made on their self-care and the care of the patient. The awareness of the American consumers' use of CAM and their desire for holistic practitioners was further fuel for the transformation of faculty to perceive the importance of the incorporation of the many aspects of holistic nursing in all courses.

Holistic nursing is presented in an orderly progression in the curriculum. During the first course, first semester, freshman year, students are introduced to the curriculum and its holistic strength. Self-care for success as a student and as a nurse is emphasized at the very beginning of the curriculum. Freshman year, the students are introduced to the broad concepts of

NURS 451	NURS 460	NURS 463	NURS 465	NURS 466	NURS 468	NURS 469	NURS 470	NURS 471	NURS 472	NURS 473	NURS 498
1,2,4,7,8,10	—	—	1	—	2	8	6	—	—	—	1,2,3,4,5
2,7,9	2	—	1	—	1,2,4	6	—	1	—	—	4
3,4,5,6,8,9	1	3	2	1,5	11–6	5,7	—	—	1,3,4,6	1,3,4,6	3
3,6,7,9,10	1,3	2	—	—	1–6	—	3	2	2,3	2,3	3
2,3,5	—	3	2,3,5	3,5	1–6	—	6	2	3,7	3,7	—
2,3,5,8,9	—	—	—	—	1–6	—	—	3	—	1,4	—
2,3,5	—	2	3	—	1–6	—	—	—	4,5,7	4,5,7	—
2,3,5,9	—	2,3	4	2,3,4	1–6	7	2	2	3,5	3,5	—
2,5,9	1,2,3	—	3	—	1–6	—	—	—	1,4	1,2,6	—
1–4	1,2,3	2	7	—	1,4	1,2	4,5	4,5	1,5	1,5	2
3,5,9	1,3	2	1	—	2	—	—	—	1,2,6	1,2,6	2
1,2,8	—	—	7	—	1–6	—	—	—	2,5	2,5	—

the holistic core through their first two courses. With each succeeding course, time is spent in integrating the core and standards as related to the specific focus of the course. Each course description clearly identifies the aspects of holistic nursing to be highlighted in the course. The clarity and inclusiveness of the course descriptions make it apparent what holistic content is to be emphasized and assist faculty in determining the focus of the course. Box 3 gives examples of holistic content found in specific courses. Every course covers specific items found in the Core Values and Standards. At the completion of the program, every core and standard has been discussed.

The holistic resources at XU include full- and part-time faculty who are committed to holistic nursing, two certified holistic nurses, and a third

Box 3. Holistic components identified in course descriptions

Nurs130 Ways of Knowing
Holism philosophy that emanated directly from Florence Nightingale
Discipline of holistic nursing practice
Nurse as an instrument of healing

Nurs132 Health and Culture
Cultural diversity and care and magico-religious traditions
Health–wellness–disease–illness
Psychophysiology of body, mind, spiritual healing

Nurs224 Nursing Therapeutics I
Holistic assessment
Spiritual development across the life span
Lifestyle patterns and habits that maintain healthy living
Emphasis on the client as an active partner in the healing process
Attentiveness to one's spirit
Transpersonal human caring and healing
Complementary/alternative therapies

Nurs225 Nursing Therapeutics I Practicum
Holistic health assessment for clients across the life span
Therapeutic communication skills
Relationships and self-assessment

Nurs230 Nursing Therapeutics II
Analysis of holistic nursing therapeutics used with individuals
    experiencing transitions—integrative therapies
Research and theoretic bases for the selection of holistic
    therapeutics
Empowered decision-making

Nurs231 Nursing Therapeutics II Practicum
Holistic promotive, preventive, and interventive nursing therapeutics;
    emphasis is on the development of critical thinking through the use
    of the nursing process, self-assessment, and therapeutic
    communication

Nurs360 Adults in Transitions
Holistic nursing therapeutics
Role of the nurse in providing health counseling and education to guide
    clients in making informed choices for health care is discussed

Nurs361 Adults in Transition Practicum
Application and evaluation of holistic nursing therapeutics
Therapeutic presence
Interventions to assist clients in exploring self-awareness, spirituality,
    and personal transformation in healing

Nurs370 Introduction to Nursing Research
Analysis and use of nursing research literature to facilitate holistic
　nursing care of individuals, families, and communities
Importance of dissemination of research findings

Nurs372 Families in Transition
Holistic health outcomes for families experiencing transitions
Role of the holistic nurse as an educator, consultant, facilitator, and
　partner with the client

Nurs373 Families in Transition Practicum
Application and evaluation of promotive, preventive, and interventive
　holistic nursing

Nurs450 Mental Health Nursing
Facilitating holistic healthy outcomes in adults experiencing mental
　health–illness transitions

Nurs451 Mental Health Nursing Practicum
Application and evaluation of promotive, preventive, and interventive
　holistic nursing therapeutics

Nurs470 Community Health Nursing
The nature of ethical problems
Care of the environment
Role of holistic nursing in health care reform

Nurs471 Community Health Nursing Practicum
Application and evaluation of promotive, preventive, and interventive
　holistic nursing therapeutics to be used with communities
　experiencing transitions
Partnership role of the community as the client/teacher with the holistic
　nurse

Nurs472 Care of the Complex Client
Emphasizing the interrelatedness of the mind, body, and spirit

Nurs473 Care of the Complex Client Practicum
Holistic assessment, intervention, and evaluation
Opportunity to practice as a holistic nurse by honoring
　a client's journey through truly knowing, partnering,
　and being present with that client

Nurs498 Senior Seminar
Professional responsibilities of the holistic nurse are reviewed
Concepts emphasized relate to the nurse as an instrument of healing
　engaged in a transpersonal human caring process, self-care, care of
　the environment and the global community

Courtesy of Xavier University Department of Nursing, Cincinnati, Ohio; with
permission.

preparing to take the certification examination. There are several major health care systems in the area that incorporate holistic nursing concepts with their patient care and offer CAM. These health care systems have been very generous and make available various expert practitioners to work with the XU nursing students. The Student Nurse Association invites faculty to discuss the preparation necessary to sit for the certification examination in holistic nursing. Recently, XU received grant money to fund a center for holistic nursing. The space is that of a classroom but it offers students, faculty, and guests an opportunity to practice and experience holistic nursing.

Lessons learned

Both schools were able to work through their curricula with the assistance of committed and involved faculty. The communities of the schools were supportive in knowing and wishing to learn about holistic care and holistic interventions.

WMU had the added advantage of having a more longstanding holistic health care department in the college that already had the support of the community and the surrounding environment. Furthermore, the Fetzer Institute, with its philosophy of strong caring and commitment to holistic tenets, was a powerful force in the community for translating holistic thinking within the population. The faculty grew together in formulating its appreciation and concern for holistic principles. The community at the same time began its appreciation for relationship-centered care that provided a synchrony for the continued acceptance of holistic nursing in the evolving curriculum.

XU in some respects also evolved as a new program since it transformed from an already existing undergraduate degree program to a holistic nursing program. The faculty was willing to examine its vision and mission and recognize the community's acceptance of its holistic program. Having a graduate program also has helped Xavier promote the holistic components as fully as possible. The literature is demonstrating increased incorporation of holistic nursing in graduate and postgraduate nursing programs [37,38].

Strategies for promoting and maintaining a holistic curriculum

At the 2003 AHNA annual meeting, a focus group of nurse educators met to identify barriers to holistic nursing. The result of that session led to a manuscript that discusses strategies to eliminate or diffuse those barriers [32].

Mariano [39], one of the participants at the conference, outlined some particularly helpful strategies for guiding others who wish to include holistic nursing in their repertoire. Her suggestions are equally helpful for those identifying ways to promote holistic nursing in schools of nursing.

Speak the language of peers

Mariano suggests that holistic nurses speak the language of their peers by avoiding the use of terms that are not similar to what others use. When colleagues embrace the notion of holistic nursing, one can begin to introduce vocabulary that is related to holistic nursing, such as therapeutic presence, transpersonal caring, and being present.

Assess interest in complementary alternative modalities

Find out through discussion or formal assessment what modalities might not be acceptable to a predominant group and what modalities certain groups seem to be using. Do your homework and find out how acceptable the notion of complementary therapy use is with your colleagues. Depending on the attitude toward the use of CAM you might find that you can speak loudly about them or you might need to demonstrate some caution and speak softly. Introduce commonly accepted therapies (guided imagery, meditation, relaxation, or massage) as a beginning point to teach or simply to discuss with peers. Keep in mind, the use of CMT does not make the nurse holistic. Emphasize the "being with" the patient versus the "doing to" the patient. When interest arises in learning about these modalities, present them. Do not make the mistake of coming on too strong when others are not ready to accept your ideas or your passions.

Support research

Support research for quality health care by documenting the relationship between holistic nursing and early recovery or greater comfort. Get involved in pilot studies that examine the effects of self-care in nursing students, exercise and movement, relaxation, and healing environments. Review current research on holistic nursing and disseminate a summary of findings that can impact the teaching and nursing care of your colleagues.

Offer your services

Offer your service to others by giving presentations to nursing groups, teaching courses, and being a guest speaker for peers. Offer services to students, faculty, and staff. Set up a workshop for stress management. For example, WMU offered 15-minute massage sessions for students during exam week. Now students and faculty throughout the college look forward to that opportunity and provide testimony to the efficacy of that service in alleviating stress during that time of the semester.

Partner with others

Florence Nightingale did not do everything on her own. She networked and found leaders to listen to her and accept her ideas. Faculty who are alone need to follow Nightingale's strategy. Find a colleague who has a similar mind-set, a senior faculty member, chairperson, or dean. Use the politics of the department, college, or university. Begin to identify the importance of holistic nursing versus non-holistic nursing. You cannot do this on your own. Find someone who is like-minded on the faculty or someone you can ask for support. There might be someone in an allied discipline that is like-minded and you can join forces. You might want to begin by offering a course for students in the two ore more related disciplines [32,39].

Start with our roots—Florence Nightingale

Listen to her voice. Share her work, quote her, but be gentle. Above all, know your curriculum. If you are considering introducing or adding holistic nursing, know your philosophy and conceptual framework. Does it fit with what your university, college, or school is doing? Educators are particularly concerned about the need to cover everything nurses need to know, do, and become. They express increasing concern that adding holistic nursing is not possible because there is so much material that needs to be covered to prepare students for the national licensing examination process.

Curriculum guides

Holistic nursing principles, content, and modalities are consistent with what nursing is and should be. Knowledge of curriculum development, use of curriculum resources from the literature, and selection of appropriate consultation are critical strategies for consideration if planning for curriculum change. In addition to the guidance offered by AHNA and AHNCC in specific curriculum help, take advantage of sound curriculum development references [40–43].

Preparing new faculty

To maintain the integrity of the holistic curriculum, occasional recharging needs to take place. When new faculty members are appointed, elements of the holistic curriculum may be omitted because of unfamiliarity with underlying concepts found in the curriculum. To continue with its holistic curriculum the program must offer materials, workshops, mentoring, and networking to introduce new faculty to the curriculum. WMU faculty found monthly meetings in which each member prepared a different aspect of holistic nursing for discussion by the group one stimulating way to share the news with others. XU offers a workshop for all faculty that discusses Nightingale's work and the nature of holistic nursing before the beginning of the school year to refresh senior faculty and orient new faculty. Learning activities focused on guidelines for developing and implementing teaching strategies to assist faculty in integrating holistic nursing into their classroom courses and clinical settings are also presented. Holistic teaching resources are available for faculty in a "holistic library." Informal round tables take place in which faculty meet and discuss their use or the students' use of holistic concepts in the clinical and classroom settings.

Summary

Holistic nursing is growing in its acceptance and importance in nursing. Organizations, such as the AHNA and the AHNCC, offer resources to assist those schools that wish to incorporate essential holistic content in their curricula. The National League for Nursing and the American Association of Colleges of Nursing and their respective accrediting bodies are critical resources for assuring that curricular components meet requirements consistent with accreditation. Overcoming barriers, enlisting the advice of others, networking with like-minded schools, serving as mentors to schools who wish to adopt holistic nursing, promoting certification among faculty, and encouraging faculty to pursue their own development as individuals and groups are helpful ways to encourage others to consider ways of incorporating holistic nursing in their schools. The authors hope that sharing their stories might serve as a catalyst for considering the value and worth of incorporating holistic nursing within your own curricula.

References

[1] Watson J. The theory of human caring: retrospective and prospective. Nurs Sci Q 1997;10(1): 49–52.

[2] Astin JA. Why patients use alternative medicine: results of a national sample. JAMA 1998; 279:1548–53.

[3] Dossey BM, Dossey L. Body-mind-spirit: attending to holistic care. Am J Nurs 1998;98(8): 35–8.

[4] Fenton MV, Morris DL. The integration of holistic nursing practices and complementary and alternative modalities into curricula of schools of nursing. Altern Ther Health Med 2003;9(4):62–7.

[5] American Holistic Nurses Association. What is holistic nursing. Available at: http://ahna. org/about/whatis.html. Accessed October 16, 2006.

[6] Nightingale F. Notes on nursing. New York: Dover Publications; 1969, 1859.

[7] Nightingale F. Training of nurses and nursing the sick. In: Quain R, editor. Dictionary of medicine. 1894. Reprinted in Williamson L (ed). Florence Nightingale and the birth of professional nursing. Bristol (UK): Thoemmes Press; 1999. p. 1, 237.

[8] Nightingale F. Sick nursing and health nursing. In: Hamptom I, editor. Nursing of the sick. New York: McGraw-Hill; (Original work published 1893). p. 24–37.

[9] Selanders LC. The power of environmental adaptation. J Holist Nurs 1998;16(2):247–63.

[10] Burkhardt MA. Reflections: awakening spirit and purpose. J Holist Nurs 1998;16(2): 165–7.

[11] Bright MA. Holistic health and healing. Philadelphia: F.A. Davis Company; 2002. p. 28.

[12] Quinn J. Healing: a model for an integrative health care system. Adv Pract Nurs Q 1997;3: 1–7.

[13] Dossey L. Samueli conference on definitions and standards: working definitions and terms. Altern Ther Health Med 2003;9(3):A10–2.

[14] Jonas WB, Chez RA, Duffy B, et al. Investigating the impact of optimal healing environments. Alternative Therapies 2003;9(6):36–40.

[15] Dossey BM, Selanders LC, Beck D, et al. Florence Nightingale today. Silver Spring (MD): American Nurses Association; 2005.

[16] Nightingale F. Private note. British Library Additional Manuscripts 45844f232; 1894. p. 2.

[17] Nightingale F. Address from Miss Nightingale to the probationer nurses in the "Nightingale Fund" School at St. Thomas' Hospital and the nurses who were formerly trained there. London (UK): Spottiswoode & Co.; 1873.

[18] Slater VE, Maloney JP, Krau SD, et al. Journey to holism. J Holist Nurs 1999;17(4):365–83.

[19] Frisch NC, Dossey BM, Guzzetta CE, et al. AHNA standards of holistic nursing practice. Gaithersburg (MD): Aspen Publishers, Inc.; 2000. p. xx.

[20] Callister LC, Bond AE, Matsumura G, et al. Threading spirituality through nursing education. Holist Nurs Pract 2004;18(3):160–6.

[21] Lemmer CM. Recognizing and caring for spiritual needs of clients. J Holist Nurs 2005;23(3): 310–22.

[22] Chase SK. Response to the concept of nursing presence: state of the science. Sch Inq Nurs Pract 2001;15(4):323–7.

[23] Doona ME, Chase SK, Haggerty LA. Nursing presence: as real as a milky way bar. J Holist Nurs 1999;17(1):54–70.

[24] Rankin EA, DeLashmutt MB. Finding spirituality and nursing presence: the student's challenge. J Holist Nurs 2006;24(4):282–8.

[25] Watson J. Nursing: human science and human care. Sudbury (MA): Jones and Bartlett Publishers; 1999. p. 49.

[26] Rew L. Self-reflection: consulting the truth within. In: Dossey BM, Keegan L, Guzzetta CE, editors. Holistic nursing: a handbook for practice. 4th edition. Sudbury (MA): Jones and Bartlett; 2005. p. 429–47.

[27] O'Brien ME. Spirituality in nursing. Sudbury (MA): Jones and Bartlett Publishers; 1999.

[28] Eisenberg DM, Davis RB, Ettner SL, et al. Trends in alternative medicine use in the United States, 1990–1997. JAMA 1998;280:1569–75.

[29] Panel on definition and description, CAM Research Methodology Conference, office of alternative medicine, National Institutes of Health, Bethesda (MD), April 1995. Available at: http://nccam,nih.gov/health/whatiscam/. Accessed October 20, 2006.

[30] Caspi O, Sechrest L, Pitluck HC, et al. On the definition of complementary, alternative, and integrative medicine: societal mega-stereotypes vs. the patients' perspectives. Alternative Therapies 2003;9(6):58–62.

[31] Barnes PM, Powell-Griner E, McFann K, et al. Complementary and alternative medicine use among adults: United States. 2002. Advance data from vital and health statistics. National Center for Health Statistics; 2004. Available at: http://nccam.nih.gov/news/ camstats.htm. Accessed October 16, 2006.

[32] King MO, Gates MF. Perceived barriers to holistic nursing in undergraduate nursing programs. Explore 2006;2(4):334–8.

[33] Richardson SE. Complementary health and healing in nursing education. J Holist Nurs 2003;21(1):20–35.

[34] Reed FC, Pettigrew AC, King MO. Alternative and complementary therapies in nursing curricula. J Nurs Educ 2000;39(3):133–9.

[35] Halcón LL, Chlan LL, Kreitzer MJ, et al. Complementary therapies and healing practices: faculty/student beliefs and attitudes and the implications for nursing education. J Prof Nurs 2003;19(6):387–97.

[36] Dossey BM, Keegan L, Guzzetta CE, editors. Holistic nursing: a handbook for practice. Sudbury (MA): Jones and Bartlett Publishers; 2005.

[37] Lane P, O'Brien U, Gooney MA. The progression of holism into postgraduate curricula in critical nursing; a discussion paper. Dimensions of Critical Care Nursing 2005;24(3):131–8.

[38] Jossens MOR, Ganley BJ. Integrated health practices: development of a graduate nursing program. J Nurs Educ 2006;45(1):16–24.

[39] Mariano C. Peer to peer mentoring: collegial caring in action. Paper Presented at the Pre-Conference Workshop, mentoring and modeling: pathways to transformational learning. 24th Annual Conference of the American Holistic Nurses Association. Scottsdale; June 2004.

[40] Bevis EO, Watson J. Toward a caring curriculum: a new pedagogy for nursing. New York: National League for Nursing; 1989.

[41] Boland DL, Finke LM. Curriculum designs. In: Billings DM, Halstead JA, editors. Teaching in nursing. A guide for faculty, 2nd edition. St Louis (MO): Elsevier; 2005. p. 145–66.

[42] Boland DL. Developing curriculum, frameworks, outcomes, and competencies. In: Billings DM, Halstead JA, editors. Teaching in nursing. A guide for faculty, 2nd edition. St. Louis (MO): Elsevier; 2005. p. 167–85.

[43] Thompson JE, Kershbaumer RM, Krisman-Scott MA. Educating advanced practice nurses and midwives. From practice to teaching. New York: Springer; 2001. p. 81–92.

ELSEVIER
SAUNDERS

Nurs Clin N Am 42 (2007) 335–353

NURSING
CLINICS
OF NORTH AMERICA

Research Paradigms and Methods for Investigating Holistic Nursing Concerns

Mary Enzman Hagedorn,
PhD, RN, CNS, CPNP, AHN-BC[a],*,
Rothlyn P. Zahourek, PhD, APRN, BC, AHN-BC[b,c]

[a]Beth El College of Nursing and Health Sciences, University of Colorado at Colorado Springs,
1250 Oak Hills Drive, Colorado Springs, CO 80919, USA
[b]University of Massachusetts, School of Nursing, Amherst, MA, USA
[c]Private Practice, Holistic Psychotherapy, Amherst, MA, USA

What is holistic nursing? How does holistic nursing research inform practice? How is holistic nursing research similar to or different from nursing research? Holistic nursing claims to be a discipline focused on healing the whole person dedicated to understanding and supporting the premise of holistic health of the patient and promoting healing in practitioners, patients, families, social groups, and communities. Holistic nursing embraces a caring-healing philosophy within each patient-community encounter.

For more than 2 decades, there have been three concepts central to nursing: health, healing, and caring. In addition, healing has been a central concept in holistic nursing. Watson [1–3] combines caring and healing in a causal connection and refers to them as "caring-healing." Newman and colleagues [4] posit that nursing is caring in the human health experience. Additionally, these authors and other nursing scholars [5] contend that three paradigms are operating within nursing: the particulate-deterministic (reductionistic), interactive-integrative (totality paradigm), and unitary-transformative (simultaneity paradigm, holistic). An explication of knowledge related to caring and healing in the human health experience and in holistic nursing is affected by the individual nurse's paradigmatic stance. Although each paradigm may be an underpinning in a specific holistic nursing study and multiple perspectives are appropriate for knowledge development in holistic nursing, a unitary-transformative perspective is essential for a full explication of holistic nursing [4].

* Corresponding author.
E-mail address: mahagedorn@aol.com (M.E. Hagedorn).

0029-6465/07/$ - see front matter © 2007 Elsevier Inc. All rights reserved.
doi:10.1016/j.cnur.2007.03.004   *nursing.theclinics.com*

Early in the history of nursing, much of the research was applied and knowledge generation evolved slowly until the late 1970s and 1980s, when research increased exponentially, focusing on patient outcomes. In the 1980s and 1990s, however, research became a major force in developing scientific knowledge for nursing practice [6]. Although holistic research has increased in the past 2 decades, a paucity of holistic nursing research still exists.

Holistic nursing research is complex and focuses on healing, particularly healing of self, others, and systems at large. Furthermore, the focus of healing research is on the healing relationship [7]. Quinn and colleagues [8] stated that this healing relationship is the "quality and characteristics of interactions between a healer and healee that facilitate healing," including "empathy, caring, love, warmth, trust, confidence, credibility, honesty, expectation, courtesy, respect, and communication." According to the American Holistic Nurses Association (AHNA) [9], holistic nursing research and scholarship should assist holistic practitioners to (1) understand the human experiences of health, healing, and illness and (2) evaluate the effects of nursing actions on the client's (patient's) health, illness, and recovery.

Holistic nursing research is challenging and necessary if nurses want support in practice. Nurses need to ask how holistic nursing research is different from other forms of research, particularly that related to complementary modalities. Research supporting holistic nursing includes descriptive, explanatory, and exploratory designs as well as combined approaches, aesthetic process, or "unusual" methods and theoretic/conceptual frameworks focused on understanding the full nature of holistic nursing. This article discusses frameworks and models for conducting holistic nursing research from philosophic and theoretic perspectives. Research methods that support conducting holistic research are also discussed. Finally, examples of research within holistic nursing are shared, and future directions for holistic nursing research are discussed.

Competing paradigmatic perspectives within holistic nursing

Holistic nurses recognize two views of holism: (1) holism identifies the interrelationships of the biopsychosocial-spiritual dimensions of the person and recognizes that the whole is greater than the sum of its parts and (2) holism understands the individual as a unitary whole in mutual process with the environment. Holistic nurses respond to both views, believing that the goals of nursing can be achieved within either framework [10].

Newman and colleagues [4] offer three competing paradigmatic perspectives operating within nursing: the particulate-deterministic, interactive-integrative, and unitary-transformative. The particulate-deterministic paradigm views phenomena as isolatable and reducible and with separate and definitive properties. These phenomena are viewed as having orderly and predictable connectedness. Change is assumed to be a consequence of antecedent conditions, and if these concepts are sufficiently understood and identified, they could predict and control change in the phenomena. Relationships within and among are viewed as linear and causal. The interactive-integrative paradigm is an extension of the particulate-deterministic perspective that also considers context and experience to account for subjective data; phenomena are viewed as having multiple interrelated parts within a specific context. Thus, reality is assumed to be multidimensional and contextual. Knowledge depends on context and is relative. The unitary-transformative paradigm represents a significant perspective shift, wherein phenomena are viewed as unitary self-organized fields embedded in a larger self-organizing field and identified by pattern and interaction with the larger whole [4]. Change is increasingly complex and unpredictable. Knowledge is personal and involves pattern recognition. Subject matter for research includes thoughts, values, feelings, choices, and purpose. Inner reality depicts the reality of the whole.

Each paradigmatic perspective specifies a point of view. Research is conceptualized, and assumptions are inherent in the paradigmatic view, providing a basis for exploration and knowledge generation. The three paradigmatic views within nursing question the prevailing stance within nursing that empiric/quantitative research is the ultimate form of research informing nursing practice. Empiric research often reduces nursing phenomena into smaller constructs/concepts and variables that are controlled, manipulated, and measured to discover their effects and generalize results to a larger population. Little significance is attributed to the emotional, psychologic, spiritual, and social aspects of nursing phenomena. Qualitative research methods investigate nursing phenomena that are viewed as unitary. Through exploration and discovery, the meanings of these phenomena are realized.

Hicks and Hennessy [11] echo this concern, focusing emphasis on how experimentation has "marginalized" alternative qualitative approaches that better describe nursing situations, "seriously limit the nursing research database" as a result. Furthermore, they suggest that a more "eclectic research approach to evidence-based care is warranted" [11].

Dahlberg and Drew [12] enlarge on their 1995 article in the *Journal of Holistic Nursing* questioning the reductionistic paradigm for nursing and add five philosophic concepts that form the basis for holistic research. Openness is the central concept in the "lifeworld" paradigm and is supported by encounter, immediacy, uniqueness, and meaning. Open-mindedness, open-heartedness, phenomenologic questioning, and preunderstanding support openness [12]. Research from this view is based on phenomenologic philosophy, wherein the researcher's openness to the "phenomena of the everyday world" is essential.

Fundamental patterns of knowing and knowledge generation

At the core of knowledge generation within holistic nursing is a passion to understand healing and wholeness more fully. Carper [13] presented nursing with a description of fundamental patterns of knowing within nursing. These included empiric, ethical, personal, and aesthetic knowing. Empiric knowing represents the traditional objective, logical, and positivistic tradition of science and is committed to providing explanations for the control and measurement of specific phenomenon. The nursing profession's alignment with empiricism provides the basis of inquiry that objectifies data and provides measurement and the generalization of results. Many studies investigating the effect of specific complementary and alternative medicine (CAM) modalities fall into this category. Aesthetic knowing is the artful knowledge within nursing. Understanding and interpretation of subjective experiences and creativity within nursing are the basis of this pattern of knowing. Aesthetic knowing is abstract and defies formal description and measurement. Several nursing scholars have linked aesthetic knowing to the development of theory and research approaches that relate to holistic nursing research [14–20]. Personal knowing requires the nurse to know self. The degree to which nurses know themselves is determined by their ability to self-actualize. Movement toward knowledge of self and self-actualization requires a comfort with ambiguity and a commitment to patience and self-care. "*Personal knowing* is a commitment to authentication of relationships and a presence with others ... the enlightenment and sensitization that humans bring to genuine human interactions" [21]. Ethical knowing reflects ethical obligations in a situation or ideas about what should be done in a given situation. Through ethical knowing, the nurse comes to a realization of what is acceptable practice. Ethical knowing is more than traditional principles and codes of ethics or conduct. Ethical knowing requires openness to differences in philosophic positions [21–24]. White [25] adds sociopolitical knowing, which promotes the premise that nurses must maintain a voice for the patient and profession through active participation in social issues key to nursing practice (eg, human vulnerability, poverty, economics, environmental issues). Munhall [26] offers "unknowing" as another pattern of knowing. Unknowing captures those things that the nurse does not grasp in the moment of the encounter with the other. Further, knowledge is shaped but is not completely defined by the process by which it is created. Studies investigate "energy" phenomena and elusive aspects of holistic nursing, such as empathy [27–31], comfort [32], presence [33–35], spirituality [36,37], caring [33,38], and intentionality [7,39–41].

Narrative knowing [42,43] is an emerging way of knowing for holistic researchers. Narrative inquiry allows holistic nurses, through storytelling [44], to gain a deeper understanding of holistic processes in practice as well as the meaning of the processes from the nurse's and patient's perspectives. The storied experience also illuminates the relationship between the nurse and patient or nurse and organization [45].

Theoretic perspectives supporting holistic nursing research

Considerable research exists stating that caring, holism, and health are concepts central to nursing. In fact, Newman and colleagues [4] contend that nursing is caring in the human health experience. Integrating these theoretic perspectives, including the concept of healing, leads us to a description of the task of holistic nursing research: the examination and explication of elemental concepts within nursing, including health, caring, healing, and holism. Three central concepts within nursing—health, caring, and holism—have received concentrated attention. Health is heralded as the centerpiece of nursing knowledge since the days of Nightingale and is discussed by nursing theorists and researchers [4]. Parse [46,47] has placed an emphasis on human experience as the basis of her theory of man-living-health, rephrased later as the human becoming. Caring has also occupied a dominant position in nursing and holistic nursing literature and research. The linkage of caring and health was espoused by many nursing researchers, including (1) Leininger [48], who claimed that caring was closely linked to health and well-being; (2) Watson [1–3,40,49], who connected caring and healing in a causal connection referred to as caring-healing; and (3) Benner and Wrubel [50], who linked caring with health and well-being.

Martha Rogers [51] developed the theoretic perspective of the science of unitary human beings. In this theory, she posed a unitary view of humans and the environment as irreducible wholes. Although Rogers did not explicate a conceptualization of healing, it was clear that a unitary conceptualization of healing grounded in wholeness would require an understanding of human/environmental wholeness as unitary [52–55]. Newman [56] captures holism as "unbroken wholeness ... what is real—not the fragments we devise with our way of describing things."

So how do we integrate these specific concepts into what we study as holistic nurses? Holistic nurses could study patients and their responses to and experiences with healing, healing interventions, or healing environments. Healing relationships or individuals as systems and how each is integral to a larger social or cultural system is also a focus of study. Healing systems need further study regarding their effect on the whole person. Interventional studies of holistic interventions (eg, Therapeutic Touch, Healing Touch, Reiki, massage, aromatherapy, massage, herbs, prayer, relaxation, imagery) would also provide additional knowledge about healing and holism specifically related to nursing interventions.

Framework for holistic nursing research

Mariano [57] has developed a framework for holistic nurse researchers, providing us with four attributes of holistic scholarship: being wide awake, reflective, caring, and humorous. First, keeping ourselves wide awake includes being attentive to others and conscious of our evolving experiences, thinking about our place in humanity, being aware of encounters by which we engage within our world and structure our reality, and a way of being open to possibility. In research, being awake frames the questions we ask, allows us to ask unexplored questions, and assists us in our discovery of unique and novel understandings; thus, we become creative open scholars. A second attribute, reflectivity, closely relates critical and ethical thinking but is an introspective process, whereby one displays to self and others a thinking process, a philosophic stance, value assumptions/biases, and a decision-making process. Reflectivity provides us with clarity, preciseness, accuracy, relevancy, consistency, and fairness. Johns [58] provides a nursing practice model, the reflective practitioner, which has implications for holistic nursing research. A reflective practice has many layers, including reflection-on-experience, whereby nurses reflect on a situation or experience after the event with the intention of drawing insights that may inform their future practice; reflection-in-action, whereby the nurse pauses within a particular situation or experience to make sense of the situation and reframe the situation, proceeding toward a desired outcome; and reflection-in-the-moment, whereby the nurse is aware of the way (s)he is thinking, feeling, and responding to the unfolding moment [58]. A reflective practice model mirrors the reflective research process.

Taylor [59] introduces us to three reflective processes in nursing: technical, practical, and emancipatory. For nurses, technical reflection fits well with the evidence-based practice model, which tests the validity of long-standing procedures and seeks to replace old untested and unproven approaches. Practical reflection involves human interactions and communicative actions relating to reciprocal expectations about behavior of others. Emancipatory reflection involves interpretation of elements and how people interpret themselves in relation to roles and social obligation. Through reflection, nurses become reflective practitioners and researchers, constructing new explanations for the unique and the familiar. Reflection also provides us with ways to examine and critique the unstated or prior understandings that direct everyday repetitive actions in practice and with new ways to experience practice.

Caring, a third element of holistic research, has been discussed previously. Holistic nurses are dedicated to studying and responding to new and pressing human health care issues, and thus to moral endeavor. In an article on caring knowledge and informed moral passion, Watson [60] posited that it was not enough to be technically competent, because if knowledge is deplete of informed passion, this can lead to domination, manipulation, control, or power. Caring (informed passion), and holistic nursing, research requires intellectual humility, courage, empathy, and fair-mindedness. Clearly, "caring without scholarship can be ordinary, but scholarship with caring can be treacherous" [57].

Finally, researchers need a sense of humor, because research demands multiple tasks and holds great uncertainty. Humor is rarely mentioned within the context of research and can assist our embracing the unknown. Using various talents, activities, skills, and professional paths, holistic nurse scholars (researchers) can participate in research revealing knowledge from all these realms. Parse [61] posited that for research to be nursing research, it has to have a nursing framework and theory rather than being just nurses doing research. Multiple paradigmatic perspectives, patterns of knowing, and divergent theoretic perspectives on "what is holism" continue to exist within nursing. These issues stimulate the holistic researcher to consider and incorporate a diverse framework for planning, conducting, and interpreting research. A summary of these paradigms and patterns of knowing is presented in Fig. 1. These authors emphasize the need for the research platform within holistic nursing to have holistic theory as a basis for problem identification, chosen research methods, and interpretation of results.

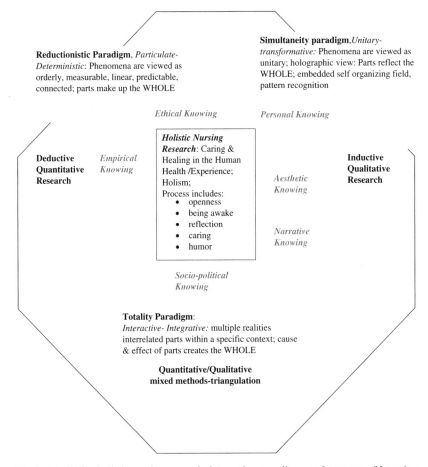

Fig. 1. Model for holistic nursing research: integrating paradigms and patterns of knowing.

All these theoretic perspectives form the framework on which holistic nursing research is conceptualized, planned, executed, and interpreted. Each has its own perspective on holism and a view of the world in which the research is conceived and fully interpreted.

Focus on holistic nursing research: changing time

Quality holistic nursing research is necessary if nurses want support in practice. Nurses need to ask how holistic nursing research is different from other forms of research, particularly those related to complementary modalities. The holistic nurse is an instrument of healing and a facilitator in the healing process. Holistic nurses honor the individual's subjective experience about health, health beliefs, and values. To become therapeutic partners with individuals, families, and communities, holistic nursing practice draws on nursing knowledge, theories, research, expertise, intuition, and creativity.

Newman [56] suggests that the prevailing holistic nursing research fails to focus on holistic commitments/principles. In an attempt to predict, control, and objectify concepts/constructs, holistic nursing has blurred nursing's paradigmatic stance of holism. In an effort to be predictive, nursing has divided the patient into parts rather than maintaining the premise of holism. With the introduction of qualitative methods in nursing more than 2 decades ago, unitary phenomena began to be investigated, patient experiences were explicated, and substantive theories emerged [52–55]. Within a philosophy of holism and healing, nurses are exploring such phenomena as presence, intuition, comfort, intention/intentionality, love, healing, spirituality, mindfulness, and compassion [7].

Holistic nurse researchers seeking to answer the questions within practice are challenged to construct knowledge that is rigorous and credible and to develop their practice and research trajectory within competing paradigms. Holistic nursing research generally evolves from three research traditions: quantitative, qualitative, and mixed methods. Creswell [62] provides a comprehensive view of these research traditions and provides a framework that is congruent with the three prevailing paradigms that Newman and colleagues [4] described as mirroring this research process: particulate-deterministic, interactive-integrative, and unitary-transformative. The knowledge claims, strategies, and methods within these views are categorized under three approaches: quantitative, qualitative, and mixed methods. In a quantitative approach, the investigator uses postpositivist/reductionistic (particulate-deterministic) claims for developing knowledge that arise from objectivity and control (eg, cause and effect, reduction of various variables, hypothesis and theory testing) as well as measurement and observation to gather data (eg, surveys, experimentation, instruments to measure variables). Alternatively, in qualitative approaches, the researcher creates knowledge claims from a subjective, unitary, experiential view based on a constructionist (unitary-transformative) perspective (eg, meanings of individual experience, meanings that are socially and historically constructed with the intent of developing a theory or pattern) or advocacy/participatory perspectives (eg, political, issue-oriented, action oriented). Qualitative research also uses aesthetic strategies of inquiry (eg, reflective journaling, photographs, art, narratives, vignettes). The researcher collects data from open-ended interviews, participant observation, and field work. Finally, in mixed methods (often referred to as triangulated), the researcher makes claims to knowledge based on pragmatic (interactive-integrative) grounds (eg, consequence-oriented, problem-centered, pluralistic). Mixed methods use strategies of inquiry that involve collecting data simultaneously or sequentially to explain research problems. Data collection involves gathering numeric information (eg, instruments, surveys) as well as textual information (structured interview formats). Research supporting holistic nursing includes methods from all three research approaches: quantitative (descriptive, correlational, and experimental), qualitative (exploratory), and mixed methods (explanatory) designs (Table 1) [63].

Within holistic nursing, several patterns of knowing support research approaches: rational/scientific, ethical, empiric, intuitive, and aesthetic. Nursing scholarship involving rational/empiric understanding is necessary to demonstrate (1) basic mechanisms of nursing actions and integrative therapies; (2) clinical safety, efficacy, and treatment outcomes of holistic modalities; and (3) the interactive nature of "bodymindspirit" [9]. Nursing research investigating the past and present experiences of the nurse and patient and research focusing on future needs and approaches of nurses and patients are the realms of holistic nursing research. Nursing scholarship involving intuitive and aesthetic understanding of phenomena and situations is necessary to comprehend dimensions of holistic work encompassing (1) the art of care, (2) the wholeness of the patient's experiences and meaning of patterns that emerge, (3) the beauty of authentic interaction, and (4) the knowledge of that which is perceived through nonverbal and nonobjective expression. These processes encompass the multiple meanings, processes, and evolving multidimensional outcomes of the caring-healing relation.

The body of knowledge that frames holistic nursing includes knowledge of the science and an understanding of the art of the profession. The AHNA supports nursing research and scholarship that builds scientific knowledge through empiric and qualitative work that extends humanistic understanding through humanistic investigations and creative expressions. The AHNA endorses nursing scholarship relevant to learning, documenting, and comprehending that which is the science and art of holistic nursing, with the goal of producing dependable and relevant information for practitioners and the public [9].

Many phenomena of concern to holistic nursing remain unknown or undocumented; thus, exploratory qualitative research methods are highly

Table 1
Guide to holistic nursing research

Paradigmatic view	Characteristics of paradigmatic view	Research methods	Description of methods
Particulate-deterministic	Views phenomena as isolatable and reducible, with separate and definitive properties Relationships are viewed as linear and causal	Quantitative methods • Descriptive • Correlational • Experimental • Quasiexperimental	Predetermined Instrument-based questions Performance data Attitude data Observational data Census data Statistical analysis
Interactive-integrative	Extension of the particulate-deterministic perspective, also taking into account the context and experience Phenomena are viewed as having multiple interrelated parts within a specific context Knowledge depends on context and is relative	Mixed methods combining quantitative and qualitative strategies	Predetermined and emerging methods Open-ended and closed-ended questions Multiple forms of data collection drawing on all possibilities Statistical and textural analysis
Unitary-transformative	Represents a significant shift in perspective in which phenomena are viewed as unitary self-organized fields embedded in a larger self-organizing field and identified by pattern and interaction with the larger whole Change is unidirectional and unpredictable	Qualitative methods • Historical research • Phenomenology • Ethnography • Grounded theory • Unitary appreciative inquiry • Philosophic inquiry • Critical social theory • Action research • Reflective practice research • Narrative inquiry • Feminist inquiry • Transpersonal research	Emerging methods Open-ended questions Interview data Observational data Document data Audiovisual data • Photographs • Artwork Text and image analysis Data generated from researcher's reflections

effective for expanding the discipline's developing body of knowledge. Further, many aspects of the human responses to health, illness, and life processes (eg, suffering, pain, compassion, spirituality) are subjective, and qualitative research methods are the most feasible way of obtaining information and understanding of the human condition. Sensitive measurement instruments that assess and document the interactive nature of each client's biologic, psychologic, emotional, sociologic, and spiritual patterns are needed as well as ongoing evaluation of nursing interventions assessing usefulness in promoting wellness and preventing illness.

Overview of holistic research studies

Research in holistic nursing has predominantly focused on the theoretic perspectives (eg, presence, empathy, spirituality, intentionality, mindfulness, reflective practice, aesthetics) and interventional studies to test CAM approaches in holistic nursing (eg, Therapeutic Touch, Reiki, reflexology, imagery). Other researchers have investigated human health experiences related to holism and healing (eg, despair, ritual, chronic illness), developed aesthetic strategies to investigate practice (eg, photography, storytelling, walking the labyrinth, life journey portraits), and provided experiential accounts of holistic nurses. Holistic nurse researchers are beginning to address the issues of practice and education as well as defining holistic modalities and experiences of nurses and patients. Research on modalities is still limited and often focused on outcome criteria regarding the benefits the specific modalities. The paucity of holistic nursing research reveals the need for ongoing definition, description, and focus for the creation of knowledge. Table 2 [64–82] provides examples of holistic research found in the literature. The table intends to be representational and not exhaustive of the extensive work in holistic nursing research that is beginning to evolve (see Table 2).

Challenges within holistic nursing research

There are many challenges for the holistic researcher. Individual, cultural, and environmental issues have an impact on the studies conducted in holistic nursing. Issues that can influence holistic nursing research include the following [7]:

1. Funding sources for studies
2. Time allotment for study
3. Interpretation and meaning of an experience
4. Other intervening life experiences
5. Environmental and cultural influences
6. Effect and timing of a specific intervention or approach, specifically placebo and experimental effects

Table 2
Examples of holistic research studies

Holistic research focus	Author	Description of study
Theoretic perspectives	Cowling, 2006 [55]	This study describes the evolution of a unitary healing praxis model derived from three unitary appreciative inquiries of despair with women. The model is based on a conceptualization of healing as appreciating the inherent wholeness of life.
	Engelbretson, 1998 [64]	The heterodox model of healing that emerged from a prior ethnographic study of healers using forms of healing touch is described, and implications for practice and research are discussed.
	Hemsley et al, 2002 [65] Taking the eagle's view: using Watson's conceptual model to investigate the extraordinary and transformative experiences of nurse healers	Watson's conceptual model of caring-healing and transpersonal understanding is used to underpin a hermeneutic-phenomenologic study of extraordinary and transformational experiences of nurse healers. The five essential themes are belonging and connecting, opening to spirit, summoning, wounding and healing journey, and living as a healer. The unity of meaning is "Walking Two Worlds."
	Zahourek, 2005 [66]	Using grounded theory methodology to develop a substantive theory of intentionality with six expert healers and six clients of the healers (healees), this study develops a conceptual framework for intentionality.
Instrument development	Delaney, 2005 [37]	A researcher-developed instrument for spirituality designed from a holistic perspective and psychometric properties was established. Three factors of spirituality are self-discovery, relationships, and eco-awareness.
	Lyin and Younger, 2005 [67]	The study describes the development and psychometric testing of an existential meaning scale.
	Rew, 2000 [68]	Development and validation of a scale to measure nurse's intuition was tested on 106 mental health nurses.
	Smith, 2006 [69]	This study describes the development and psychometric testing of an instrument to assess intuition.
Education	Delaney, 2006 [70]	Aesthetic knowing in nursing informs this pedagogic approach to educating nurses about the construct of aesthetic knowing, using a trip to the art museum as the context to provide insights about aesthetics in nursing.
	Fenton and Morris, 2006 [71]	Using an electronic Web survey, 125 deans of schools of nursing are surveyed about the integration of complementary and alternative medicine into their curricula of nursing.

Education	Sharoff, 2006 [72]	Using a qualitative naturalistic design of 10 experienced holistic nurses, this research reveals that participants described a lack of juncture between traditional nursing and their personal and professional growth and the need for credibility as key to them becoming competent practicing holistic nurses.
Practice	O'Quinn, 1995 [73]	Using a correlational design, the researcher compares work site wellness programs and behaviors of nurses.
	Enzman Hagedorn, 2005 [33]	Using poetry and story as well as Watson's 10 *caritas*, the caring practices of nurse practitioners are presented and a new philosophy for advanced practice nursing is posed that incorporates the medical model to inform patient care and the tenets of caring as an art and science to actualize nursing practice.
	Hagedorn and Quinn, 2005 [74]	Using clinical exemplars, this qualitative study describes how caring theory guides nurse practitioner practice. The attitudes of caring of nurse practitioners include connection, consistency, commitment, community, and change.
Modalities	Wardell and Engelbretson, 2001 [75]	This is a study on Reiki, using several physiologic measures to assess the effectiveness of this modality.
	Brathovde, [76]	The study uses triangulated interviews and a self-report caring scale to assess the effectiveness of Reiki as a self-care approach for nurses and health care providers.
	Hanley, 2004 [77]	Using narrative inquiry and qualitative descriptive methods, the researchers explore the nature of Therapeutic Touch with preterm infants and describe a Therapeutic Touch protocol for this vulnerable population.
	Sandor and Froman, 2006 [78]	This research describes an experimental study designed to evaluate the effectiveness of walking the labyrinth and its potential uses within practice. Although no significant findings are revealed, this study shows how complex investigating interventions for holistic nursing can be.
	Peck, 1997 [79]	This is a quantitative study designed to measure the effectiveness of Therapeutic Touch in elderly patients with generative arthritis.
	Smith et al, 2003 [80]	This is a quantitative study designed to measure the effects of Therapeutic Touch during bone marrow procedures.
	Morris, 2006 [81]	This study describes the results of a quasiexperimental pilot study of perimenopausal and postmenopausal women and their sense of relaxation after a 50-minute reflexology session once a week.

(continued on next page)

Table 2 (continued)

Holistic research focus	Author	Description of study
Aesthetics	Gaydos, 2003 [17]	The cocreative aesthetic process is presented as a new model to describe aesthetics in nursing and four aspects: engagement, mutuality, movement, and new form. This study demonstrates how the cocreative aesthetic process demonstrates a necessity for caring with holism in the art of nursing.
	Enzman Hagedorn, 1996 [20]	This study describes an aesthetic technique (hermeneutic photography) that can be used in qualitative research to capture the essence of lived experience. This technique emerged from a previous study describing the family's lived experience of childhood chronic illness [18].
	Mitchell, and Halifax, 2005 [82]	This study discusses a phenomenologic study based on Parse's human becoming theory that used art to gather the experience of feeling respected or not respected for a community of artists.

7. Personal experience and problems that arise for the researcher
8. Personality, belief systems, spiritual practices, and temperament of the researcher and participant
9. Difficulty in trying to standardize modalities, variations in methods, and approach and skill of the researcher
10. Influence of studying a phenomenon or person within a naturalistic setting
11. Interpretation of results
12. Recognized value of qualitative and quantitative results
13. Importance of the relationship between the healer and the one being healed

Clarity of what is meant by holism and unitary and how terms are used in a proposed study is essential. When conducting a quantitative study, the researcher needs to consider confounding variables and to select methods, techniques, and tools that are in concert with the variables being studied. The outcome measures should be operationally defined and clearly articulated in the study.

Individual scholars and groups, such as the Samueli Group [83], recommend the use of mixed methods that include qualitative approaches. Scholars are cautioned that qualitative data of a few add-on "qualitative" questions are not necessarily legitimate qualitative data. Researchers need to be familiar with the complexity of the selected method. All forms of data collection may be enlivened by the careful addition of creative data collection and analysis incorporating poetry, dance, song, photography, art, and journaling. The researcher needs to anticipate the multiple challenges that holistic nursing research presents.

Funding for holistic research provides one of the largest challenges for researchers. The national platforms provide limited research funding to researchers, and this funding is extremely competitive. The National Institute for Nursing Research (NINR) funds only a limited number of submitted proposals, and quantitative studies are funded more often than qualitative studies. The AHNA has developed small grant funding for research conducted by its members. The challenge to the holistic researcher is to tap multiple sources for the funding of projects. Foundations, private industry, and other resources for funding need to be explored and developed.

Preparing the proposal of the research is a first step. Frisch and colleagues [84] have provided guidelines for preparing holistic research proposals. When presenting a proposal for funding of a research project, the researcher must convince the funding source that he or she is knowledgeable about the topic, able to implement the proposed study, and competent to carry out all aspects of the research design. The goal for a holistic nursing researcher is to present a well-balanced and sound proposal that clearly defines the study and its importance to the field of holistic nursing.

Future of holistic nursing research

This article has presented multiple ideas that are key to the success of conducting holistic nursing research. The challenge is to conduct research that is focused on a clear definition of "holism," uses holistic theory to frame the study, and uses a method that is focused on creating new knowledge and theoretic perspectives within holistic nursing. Holistic nurse researchers need to provide credible and reliable results that can direct activities within practice, education, or future research. Many concepts within nursing have yet to be thoroughly defined or researched (eg, compassion, ritual, presence). Few studies have been conducted to evaluate the effectiveness of CAM activities within nursing practice. Many modalities are being used without explanation of the benefits or risks related to these modalities. The key issues to address in holistic nursing research include finding a relevant and researchable holistic nursing question, providing evidence to answer the research question and, finally, evaluating and summarizing the worth of the findings to holistic nursing. Clinicians need to apply results and evaluate the process and interventions that emerge from studies. This process must be constantly nurtured by the practice arena.

The primary goal of holistic nursing research is to develop and expand the knowledge base of holism and healing for education and practice. As more holistic researchers emerge wanting to study concepts within holistic nursing, the challenges of holistic research are likely to be realized. Future knowledge is likely to be shaped by the research presently being conducted. Holistic nurse researchers are likely to conduct research based on their paradigmatic views and are challenged to be rigorous about the process. New knowledge is waiting to be revealed by holistic researchers. Researchers are mandated to begin to build methods that are grounded in personal epistemologic foundations, adhere to systematic reasoning of the discipline of nursing, and yield legitimate knowledge for practice [85]. Research testing CAM effects, developing theoretic explanations for holistic phenomena, and descriptions of experiences of nurses and patients interacting within the human health experience are ground for future studies. "A discipline is distinguished by a domain of inquiry that represents a shared belief among its members regarding its reason for being" [4].

References

[1] Watson J. New dimensions of human caring theory. Nurs Sci Q 1988;1:175–81.
[2] Watson J. Postmodern nursing and beyond. New York (NY): Harcourt-Brace; 1999. p. 1–152.
[3] Watson J. Caring science as sacred science. Philadelphia (PA): FA Davis Company; 2005.
[4] Newman M, Sime A, Corcoran-Perry S. The focus of the discipline of nursing. ANS Adv Nurs Sci 1991;14(1):1–6.
[5] Fawcett J. Analysis and evaluation of nursing theories. Philadelphia: FA Davis Co; 1993.

[6] Burns N, Groves S. The practice of nursing research: conduct, critique, and utilization. St. Louis (MO): Elsevier; 2005.

[7] Zahourek R. What is holistic nursing research? Is it different? Beginnings 2006;26(5): 4–6.

[8] Quinn J, Smith M, Rittenbaugh C, et al. Research guidelines for assessing the impact of healing relationship in clinical nursing. Definitions and standards in healing research. Altern Ther Health Med 2003;9(3 Suppl):A65–79.

[9] AHNA. AHNA position statements. 2003; Available at: www.ahna.org. Accessed November 26, 2006.

[10] AHNA. What is holistic nursing? 2004; Available at: www.ahna.org. Accessed November 26, 2006.

[11] Hicks C, Hennessy D. Mixed messages in nursing research: their contribution to the persisting hiatus between evidence and practice. J Adv Nurs 1997;24(3):595–601.

[12] Dahlberg K, Drew N. A lifeworld paradigm for nursing research, 1997. J Holist Nurs 1997; 15(3):3303–7.

[13] Carper B. Fundamental patterns of knowing in nursing. ANS Adv Nurs Sci 1978;1(13): 13–23.

[14] Butcher C. The unitary field pattern portrait research method: facets, processes, and findings. Nurs Sci Q 2005;1(4):293–7.

[15] Chinn P, Kramer M. Integrated knowledge development in nursing. St. Louis (MO): Mosby; 2004. p. 193–217.

[16] Gaydos HL. "Making special" a framework for understanding the art of holistic nursing. J Holist Nurs 2004;22(2):152–63.

[17] Gaydos HL. The cocreative aesthetic process: a new model for aesthetics in nursing. International Journal for Human Caring 2003;7(3):40–4.

[18] Enzman Hagedorn M. A way of life: a new beginning each day. The family's lived experience of childhood chronic illness. 1993; [doctoral dissertation]. University of Colorado, Denver (CO). University Microfilms International No. 9324737.

[19] Enzman Hagedorn M. Hermeneutic photography: an innovative aesthetic technique for generating data in nursing research. ANS Adv Nurs Sci 1994;17(1):44–50.

[20] Enzman Hagedorn M. Photography: an aesthetic technique for nursing inquiry. Issues Ment Health Nurs 1996;17:517–27.

[21] Gadow S. Existential advocacy: philosophical foundation of nursing. In: Spicker S, Gadow S, editors. Nursing: images and ideals. New York (NY): Springer; 1988.

[22] Gadow S. Ethical narrative in practice. Nurs Sci Q 1996;9(1):8–9.

[23] Kostas-Polston EA, Hayden SJ. Living ethics: contributing to knowledge through building qualitative inquiry. Nurs Sci Q 2006;19(4):304–10.

[24] Peter E. The interplay between the abstract and the particular: research ethics standards and the practice of research as symbolic. Nurs Sci Q 2006;19(1):20–4.

[25] White J. Patterns of knowing: review, critique, and update. ANS Adv Nurs Sci 1995;17: 73–86.

[26] Munhall P. Unknowing: toward another pattern of knowing in nursing. Nurs Outlook 1993; 41:125–8.

[27] Kunyk D, Olson J. Clarification of conceptualizations of empathy. J Adv Nurs 2001;35(3): 317–23.

[28] Yegdich T. On the phenomenology of empathy in nursing: empathy or sympathy? J Adv Nurs 1999;30(1):83–93.

[29] Reynolds W, Scott B. Empathy: a crucial component of the helping relationship. J Psychiatr Ment Health Nurs 1999;6:363–70.

[30] Reynolds W, Scott B, Jessiman W. Empathy has not been measured in clients' terms or effectively taught: a review of the literature. J Adv Nurs 1999;30(5):1177–85.

[31] Reynolds W, Scott P, Austin W. Nursing, empathy and perception of the moral. J Adv Nurs 2000;32(1):235–42.

[32] Kolcaba K. Comfort as process and product, merged in holistic nursing art. J Holist Nurs 1995;13(2):117–31.

[33] Enzman Hagedorn M. Caring practices in the 21st century: the emerging role of nurse practitioners. Topics in Advanced Practice Nursing eJournal 2005;4(4):22–37.

[34] Godkin J. Healing presence. J Holist Nurs 2001;19(1):5–21.

[35] Osterman P, Schwartz-Barcott D. Presence: four ways of being there. Nurs Forum 1997; 31(2):23–30.

[36] Burkhardt M, Nagai-Jacobson M. Spirituality: living our connectedness. (NY): Delmar Thomson Learning; 2002.

[37] Delaney C. The spirituality scale. Development and psychometric testing of a holistic instrument to assess the human spiritual dimension. J Holist Nurs 2005;23(2):143–67.

[38] Appleton C. The art of nursing: the experience of patients and nurses. J Adv Nurs 1993;18: 892–5.

[39] Pilkington F. The concept of intentionality in human science nursing theories. Nurs Sci Q 2005;18(2):98–104.

[40] Watson J. Intentionality and caring-healing consciousness: a practice of transpersonal nursing. Holist Nurs Pract 2002;16(4):12–9.

[41] Zahourek R. Intentionality forms the matrix for healing: a theory. Altern Ther Health Med 2004;10(6):40–9.

[42] Connelly F, Clandinin D. Stories of experience and narrative inquiry. Educational Research 1990;9:2–14.

[43] Polkinghorne D. Narrative knowing and the human sciences. Albany (NY): State of New York University Press; 1988.

[44] Sandelowki M. Truth/story telling in nursing inquiry. In: Kikuchi JF, Simmons H, Romyn D, editors. Truth in nursing inquiry. Beverly Hills (CA): Sage; 1996. p. 111–24.

[45] Hanley M. Therapeutic touch with preterm infants: composing a treatment [doctoral dissertation]. University of Texas Medical Branch, Galveston, UMI CINAHL, AN: 2005090428; 2004.

[46] Parse R. Man-living-health: a theory of nursing. New York (NY): John Wiley; 1981.

[47] Parse R. The human becoming school of thought: a perspective for nurses and other health professionals. Thousand Oaks (CA): Sage Publications; 1998.

[48] Leininger M. The essence of nursing and health. Thorofare (NJ): Slack Publishing; 1984.

[49] Watson J. Nursing. The philosophy and science of caring. Boston: Little Brown, and Company; 1979.

[50] Benner P, Wrubel J. The primacy of caring. San Francisco (CA): Addison-Wesley; 1989.

[51] Rogers M. An introduction in the theoretical basis of nursing. Philadelphia (PA): FA Davis; 1970.

[52] Cowling WR. Healing as appreciating wholeness. ANS Adv Nurs Sci 2000;22(3):16–32.

[53] Cowling WR. Unitary appreciative inquiry. ANS Adv Nurs Sci 2001;23(4):32–48.

[54] Cowling WR. Despair: a unitary appreciative inquiry. ANS Adv Nurs Sci 2004;27(4): 287–300.

[55] Cowling WR. A unitary healing praxis model for women in despair. Nurs Sci Q 2006;19(2): 123–32.

[56] Newman M. Experiencing the whole. ANS Adv Nurs Sci 1997;20(1):34–9.

[57] Mariano C. The many faces of scholarship. Beginnings 2006;26(5):3–18.

[58] Johns C. Becoming a reflective practitioner. Oxford (UK): Blackwell Publishing; 2005.

[59] Taylor B. Technical, practical, and emancipatory reflection for practicing holistically. J Holist Nurs 2004;22(1):73–84.

[60] Watson J. Caring knowledge and informed moral passion. ANS Adv Nurs Sci 1990;13(1): 15–24.

[61] Parse R. What constitutes nursing research. Nurs Sci Q 2003;16(4):281–7.

[62] Creswell J. Research design. Qualitative, quantitative and mixed methods approaches. 2nd edition. (CA): Sage Publications; 2003. p. 37–42.

[63] Speziale Streubert H, Rinaldi Carpenter D. Qualitative research in nursing. Advancing the humanistic imperative. 3rd edition. Philadelphia (PA): Lippincott, Williams & Wilkins; 2003.

[64] Englebretson J. A heterodox model of healing. Altern Ther Health Med 1998;4(2):37–42.

[65] Hemsley M, Glass N, Watson J. Taking the eagle's view: using Watson's conceptual model to investigate the extraordinary and transformative experiences of nurse healers. Holist Nurs Pract 2002;20(2):85–94.

[66] Zahourek R. Intentionality: evolutionary development in healing: a grounded theory study for holistic nursing. J Holist Nurs 2005;23(1):89–109.

[67] Lyin DE, Younger S. Development and preliminary evaluation of the existential meaning scale. J Holist Nurs 2005;23(1):54–65.

[68] Rew L. Acknowledging intuition in clinical decision making. J Holist Nurs 2000;18(2): 94–108.

[69] Smith AJ. Continued psychometric evaluation of an intuition instrument for nursing students. J Holist Nurs 2006;24(2):82–90.

[70] Delaney C. A trip to the art museum as a pedagogical approach to the teaching-learning of nursing aesthetics with RN-to-BSN student. J Nurs Educ 2006;45(3):143–4.

[71] Fenton M, Morris D. Integration of holistic nursing practices and complementary and alternative modalities into curricula of schools of nursing. Altern Ther Health Med 2006;9(4): 62–7.

[72] Sharoff L. A qualitative study of how experienced certified holistic nurses learn to become competent practitioners. J Holist Nurs 2006;24(2):116–24.

[73] O'Quinn J. Worksite wellness programs and lifestyle behaviors. J Holist Nurs 1995;13(4): 346–60.

[74] Hagedorn S, Quinn A. Theory-based nurse practitioner practice: caring in action. Topics in advanced practice nursing eJournal 2005;4(4):10–21.

[75] Wardell D, Engebretson J. Biological correlates of Reiki touch healing. J Adv Nurs 2001; 33(4):439–45.

[76] Brathovde A. A pilot study of Reiki for self care of nurses and healthcare providers. Holist Nurs Pract 2006;20(2):95–101.

[77] Hanley MA. Therapeutic touch with preterm infants: composing a treatment [abstract]. Visions: Journal of Society of Rogerian Scholars 2004;12(1):64–5.

[78] Sandor M, Froman R. Exploring the effects of walking the labyrinth. J Holist Nurs 2006; 24(2):103–10.

[79] Peck S. The effectiveness of therapeutic touch for decreasing pain in elders with degenerative arthritis. J Holist Nurs 1997;15(2):176–98.

[80] Smith M, Reeder F, Daniel L, et al. Outcomes of therapeutic touch during bone marrow transplant. Altern Ther Health Med 2003;9(1):40–9.

[81] Morris D. Pilot study using reflexology. Beginnings 2006;26(5):28–9.

[82] Mitchell G, Halifax N. Feeling respected-not respected: the embedded artist in Parse method research. Nurs Sci Q 2005;18(2):105–12.

[83] O'Malley P. Studying optimal healing environments: challenges and proposals. J Altern Complement Med 2005;11(1):S17–22.

[84] Frisch N, Rew L, Enzman Hagedorn M. Guidelines for preparing research proposals. Beginnings 2006;26(5):20–2.

[85] Thorne S, Kirkham S, McDonald-Emes J. Interpretive description: a noncategorical qualitative alternative for developing nursing knowledge. Res Nurs Health 1997;20:169–77.

ELSEVIER
SAUNDERS

NURSING
CLINICS
OF NORTH AMERICA

Nurs Clin N Am 42 (2007) 355–360

Index

Note: Page numbers of article titles are in **boldface** type.

Moving?

Make sure your subscription moves with you!

To notify us of your new address, find your **Clinics Account Number** (located on your mailing label above your name), and contact customer service at:

E-mail: elspcs@elsevier.com

800-654-2452 (subscribers in the U.S. & Canada)
407-345-4000 (subscribers outside of the U.S. & Canada)

Fax number: 407-363-9661

Elsevier Periodicals Customer Service
6277 Sea Harbor Drive
Orlando, FL 32887-4800

*To ensure uninterrupted delivery of your subscription, please notify us at least 4 weeks in advance of move.

ELSEVIER